LEARNING MEDICINE 1995

LEARNING MEDICINE 1995

AN INFORMAL GUIDE TO A CAREER IN MEDICINE

PETER RICHARDS MA MD PhD FRCP

with drawings by Paul Cox

Published by the BMJ Publishing Group
Tavistock Square, London WC1H 9JR

First edition 1983
Second edition 1985
Third edition 1986
Fourth edition 1987
Fifth edition 1988
Sixth edition 1989
Seventh edition 1990
Eighth edition 1991
Ninth edition 1992
Tenth edition 1993
Eleventh edition 1994

ISBN 0 7279 0890 1

Made and printed in England by
Latimer Trend & Company Ltd, Plymouth

The Liberty of our Commonwealth is most infringed by three sorts of men, Priests, Physicians and Lawyers. The one deceives men in matters belonging to their souls, the other in matters belonging to their bodies, and the third in matters belonging to their estates.   SAMUEL HARTLIB (seventeenth century)

... what is not negotiable is that our profession exists to serve the patient, whose interests come first. None but a saint could follow this principle all the time; but so many doctors have followed it so much of the time that the profession has been generally held in high regard. Whether its remedies worked or not, the public have seen medicine as a vocation, admirable because of the doctor's dedication.   SIR THEODORE FOX (1976)

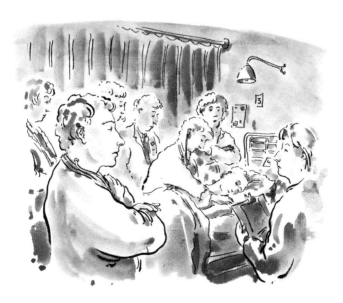

Preface to eleventh edition

This book was written to help those considering a career in medicine to discover what medicine and a medical education is all about. It was also designed to help them develop their own ideas and make their own decisions.

A schoolboy reviewer once criticised *Learning Medicine* for lacking enthusiasm. In fact my enthusiasm for a career second to none has been deliberately controlled to avoid stirring up unrealistic expectations. In the past years there has been vociferous criticism that entrants know too little about what they are letting themselves in for with the result that some doctors are disillusioned later. In my view bright eyes are not easily dulled nor do I wish to extinguish their sparkle—only to ensure that, as far as is possible, commitment is informed and realistic, not least for women and mature students.

Much is changing rapidly: undergraduate medical courses are becoming more integrated, specialist postgraduate education is being shortened, and the very structure of health care itself is in transition. Many details are uncertain but the general picture can now be painted. Change is painful but by the time those starting to learn medicine today qualify, most of the turmoil should be over and some of the benefits should have been achieved; at least junior doctors should be getting a better deal. Whatever the shape and colour of health care tomorrow, high standards of medical practice will still be central to human happiness.

PETER RICHARDS
Pro Rector (Medicine)
Imperial College
Dean and Professor of Medicine
St Mary's Hospital Medical School
University of London
1994

Contents

Why medicine and why not?

... the conviction that the medical profession as it might be was the finest in the world; presenting the most perfect interchange between science and art; offering the most direct alliance between intellectual conquest and the social good.

GEORGE ELIOT *Middlemarch*

There is a stereotype that a doctor is giving and caring, but I think those who are married to their careers are probably very selfish, with nothing to give, emotionally, to anything else.

A RECENT, DISTINGUISHED GRADUATE (1991)

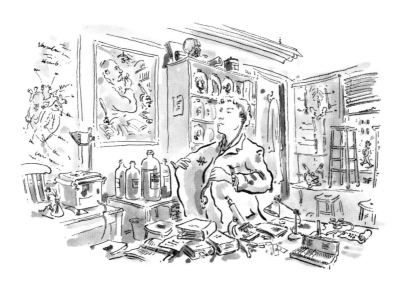

Medicine is a degree course with a difference, partly because most of those who embark on it will one day be let loose on the public as doctors, and partly because it is one of the longest and certainly the most expensive course of study. The medical course not only teaches one how to think and to reason within medicine but should also be a key to much wider understanding. Medicine is in fact no

Why medicine and why not?

bad training for life but at a cost of about £150 000 over five years it is far too precious a national investment to be used purely as general education.

Why should so many school leavers, some of those finishing another degree course, and even those already established in a different career consider becoming doctors? A desire to help people is often given as a reason. But do not policemen, porters, and plumbers of sympathetic disposition do that? It surely is not necessary to become a doctor to help people. If more pastoral care is in mind why not become a priest, a social worker, or a school teacher? If a curing edge on caring is the attraction remember that doctors do not always cure. Better perhaps to become a pharmacologist developing new drugs rather than a jobbing doctor. Also understand that the cost of attempting to cure, whether by drugs or by knife, is sometimes to make worse. A doctor must accept and live with uncertainty and fallibility, inescapable parts of any walk of life but harder to bear in matters of life or death.

A love of meeting people is another common plea. Much nearer the mark was the applicant at interview who said, "I like people," then paused and added, "Well, I don't like them all but I find them all interesting." Success in many walks of life depends on an ability to communicate with all sorts of individuals. A doctor can become a trusted friend to very different people; doctors have the privilege of a passport to rich and poor alike. Unfortunately the practical domestic difficulties of one doctor providing continuity of care by day, by night, and at weekends and, in large cities, to a constantly changing population, are to some extent eroding the special relationship between doctor and patient.

An interest in how the body works in health or in disease itself often points to a career in medicine. The former interest might, however, best be served by becoming an anatomist or physiologist and devoting oneself to a lifetime study of the structure and function of the body. As for disease itself, many scientists study aspects of disease processes without having medical qualifications. Many more people are curious about how the body works than either wish to or can become doctors.

More earthy considerations motivate many, although few are prepared to admit as much. Medicine has an "up market" image, a social accolade; entry to medicine is often seen by parents, if not by their children, as the foot of a ladder leading to social advancement. Even schoolteachers are not always above pushing a pupil towards medicine because of the reflected glory of sending students to much sought after medical schools year by year—poor but inescapable reasons these. No less earthy but possibly less generative of stress is the simple search for a job which is both relatively secure and well paid. Many other careers are more or less as secure and well paid and in some respects less demanding. Nevertheless, medicine does offer a good and secure living and who knows whether an initially pragmatic motive prevents the emergence of a good doctor? A desire for job satisfaction is often expressed at interview. Any job well done should give great satisfaction so this seems to be an insufficient reason of itself. Medicine is, however, favoured in that the routine is never without refreshing variety—the variety which is an inescapable part of mankind and womankind. Further, medicine is undoubtedly attractive as a springboard to very wide career opportunities, dealing with patients or not, as the case may be, and undertaking tasks which by and large are worldwide in their application. An international market still exists for medical graduates, albeit a shrinking one. But medicine is not unique because the world also beckons to engineers, scientists, lawyers, teachers, and nurses, to mention only a few.

Sometimes the reasons for considering medicine as a career are more personal, such as illness in the family, which has shown how much can be done to relieve suffering and anxiety, or disability such as mental handicap, which has shown how those affected can be helped to make the most of their abilities.

To be ill oneself is such a revealing experience that it prompted F J Ingelfinger, editor of the *New England Journal of Medicine*, then near the point of death himself, to write:

> In medical school, students are told about the perplexity, anxiety and misapprehension that may affect the patient ... and in the clinical years the fortunate and sensitive student may learn much from talking to those assigned to his supervision. But the effects of lectures and conversations are ephemeral and are no substitute for actual experience. One might suggest, of course, that only those who have been hospitalised during their adolescent or adult years be admitted to medical school. Such a practice would not only increase the number of empathic doctors; it would also permit the whole elaborate system of medical school admissions to be jettisoned.

Few would accept personal experience of illness as the sole qualification for entry to medical school but as a supplementary qualification it has much to recommend it.

Some are drawn to medicine by the personal influence of a sympathetic local doctor or a medical relative. Admiration alone may be a slender reason for career choice, but when admiration is tempered with critical insight into what the job demands the reason is convincing. Doctors' children have a readily available opportunity to discover what medicine is about (although some do not take the trouble to find out). At the same time there is a danger that their career choice may simply represent the tramlines of unthinking predestination or the lure of easy entry into a thriving

Why medicine and why not?

family business. At worst, a medical parent may exert pressure, a potentially deeply damaging influence on which Henry Fielding in *Tom Jones* blamed the failings of Dr Blifil, "a gentleman who had the misfortune of losing the advantage of great talents by the obstinacy of his father, who would breed him to a profession he disliked . . . the doctor had been obliged to study physick, or rather to say that he had studied it. . ."

All said and done, if you have decided on a career in medicine but cannot give a clear and convincing reason why, you should be neither upset nor too surprised.

Many doctors are unclear why they embarked on their career. Few finally regret their decision but many have misgivings in their early postgraduate years.

While a wise and clever head is necessary for medicine, sharp eyes, perceptive hearing, and a safe pair of hands are invaluable. A large part of the satisfaction in many branches of medicine derives from practical tasks well done. Practical skills tend to be undervalued both by potential applicants themselves and perhaps by selectors for entry to medicine.

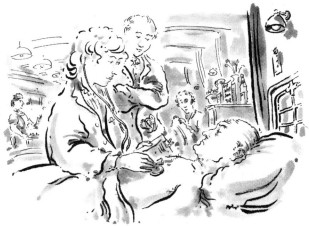

Reasons against reading medicine are not difficult to find. The course lasts five or six years; it is concentrated and sometimes dull, especially in the early years, when the emphasis tends to be on teaching endless facts rather than on learning a method of approach and reasoning. Both the training and the job itself are physically and emotionally taxing, partly because of long hours but especially because of exposure to illness, death, and dying. Becoming a doctor will not necessarily bring you unstinted admiration, partly because public regard for doctors is quietly ebbing as the mystique of medicine is gradually eroded by newspapers, books, radio, and television and partly because increasing litigation makes medical practice more prone to bad publicity. Patients are becoming more critical of the quality of their medical care and quicker to sue for alleged negligence.

Both intending applicants and selection panels need to remember that the medical course is a preparation for clinical responsibility and not only an academic degree course. The ability to pass school examinations is only one credential for acceptance, necessary but not all important. Once a doctor has qualified the early years of his or her career are more physically demanding than most, entailing long hours of work by day, by night, and at weekends and the strain of unaccustomed responsibility for the lives of others. Perhaps most constraining of all is the fact that a further five to 10 years of postgraduate training lie ahead after qualification. This training involves obtaining a series of posts, in open competition and often in different parts of the country. Settling down and getting on with family life may be difficult and for women brings the additional conflict between career and starting a family, especially if married to a doctor whose own career may develop in different directions (see the chapter on Opportunity and fulfilment, page 14). Some doctors manage to separate their private lives and hobbies from their work, but for most medicine dominates their lives and those of their families.

In addition to the stress and strain of the work itself, there is anxiety that posts are becoming harder to get as the number of graduates increases; enough training posts do exist but vacancies may not be where one wishes or in the specialty of first choice. Serious attempts are now being made nationally to ensure that all training posts lead to permanent posts within a reasonable space of time. Contrary to rumour there is no convincing evidence that many doctors will be unemployed. Employment prospects remain better in medicine than in most other professions but much greater flexibility in choice of specialty and in location of living will be required in the future than has been customary in the past.

Hours of work are still generally very long and working conditions poor, especially in hospitals. Prospects for a better career structure and shorter hours are improving but the demands in medicine will always be heavier than in most professions and more disruptive of private life.

The confidence of others, regardless of wealth or poverty or social position, is a privilege; the opportunity to understand and to help, if not to cure, is an even greater privilege. Fancy is often more frightening than fact; the doctor has to reduce fears to facts and then to set about putting things as right as is possible. Medicine is no career for the faint hearted, nor for the weak in health, nor for complainers or clock watchers. Yet for all its demands it offers the opportunity of a deeply satisfying lifetime of service to those prepared to give themselves to it.

Opportunity and fulfilment

For a start, let's bury the idea that male and female students have different aspirations – we all wish to end up well-rounded human beings . . .

THREE ST GEORGE'S MEDICAL STUDENTS (1993)

Medicine is a most suitable career for intelligent educated women who aspire to married life because it carries far more opportunities for flexible working than other professions . . . My message is: remember, women have struggled for centuries to have lives of their own and to be defined in terms of their own achievements, not someone else's.

SUSAN M ANDREW (1993)

Regrettably, but perhaps inevitably, life is not equal and medicine is no exception. To some extent inequality in medicine stems from the long and unsocial hours of work but it may also be coloured by traditional attitudes of the profession. Inequality also reflects educational opportunity and attitudes and conventions of the community, a community which in the UK is more constraining to the professional fulfilment of women than in North America and Northern Europe. Quality of school education, career horizons, gender, race and age all come into the picture. Medical connections were once an advantage but are no longer, except to the extent that it should be easier to find out what medicine is about. About one fifth of both applicants and entrants to medicine have a medical parent.

The overwhelming preponderance of applications to learn medicine from the professional and clerical sections of society partly reflects a widespread belief among others that they would not stand a fair chance of acceptance by a medical school and that, if accepted, they might not in due course fit happily into what is often seen as, and may in fact often be, a stereotyped profession. Reluctance to apply also reflects social pressures to conform to the traditional patterns of employment of any particular section of society, and a degree of social immobility imposed by peer-pressure which may be stronger within indigenous than immigrant communities. A decision not to take up medicine may also reflect financial pressures from family or friends to earn as soon as possible, together with relative inability or unwillingness to withstand the economic hardship of a long university course, especially as student support grants continue to decline in real value. Most medical schools are very keen to widen the social and cultural spectrum of their students and no one should feel inhibited from applying because of an unconventional background.

When corrected for academic attainment, personal characteristics, and evidence of commitment to a medical career, there is currently no evidence that social class, age, gender or type of school influences the chances of selection for medicine. Academic achievement counts most in short-listing for interview, but at interview non-academic factors are more important, because all applicants are apparently more than adequate academically. The non-academic factors concerned fall into two broad groups—wider interests and community service. It could of course be that a measure of discrimination, justified or not according to your point of view, derives from the fact that some sections of the community may be better placed than others to develop wider interests and caring responsibilities. Few, however, would deny that it is both logical and desirable to look for more than narrow scholastic achievement. Whether, taking all these considerations into account, any particular group is otherwise disadvantaged—for example, by race or colour—is uncertain but there are indications that ethnic minority groups may be. One study published in 1989 predicted acceptance rates for home students on objective assessment of their application forms alone as 47.8% for white students and 35.6% for ethnic minority groups compared with actual acceptance rates of 49.6% and 27.3%, respectively. The study did not determine whether the difference was in short-listing or in the outcome of interview. Later, when applying for junior hospital doctor posts, British graduates with non-European names took longer to get short-listed for interview, although once short-listed they were not at a disadvantage. Likewise a more recent study in which identical curriculum vitae were submitted under different names for hospital posts showed that an applicant bearing a European name was more likely to be short-listed.

Women have equal opportunity for entry to medicine. The days in which women were discriminated against by a quota have passed and career advisers are less discouraging, at least on the grounds of "you won't get in", although they may now not unreasonably be concerned about the much publicised difficulties of junior doctors. Women now apply in fractionally larger numbers than men and are marginally more successful in gaining acceptance. In 1992/93 50.2% of applicants and 52.1% of those accepted to study medicine at a UK university were women. Women achieve higher academic results in university entrance generally than men, although this is not reflected subsequently in higher degree class; degree class cannot be correlated in medicine, in finals at least, because it is a pass/fail examination. At interview 18 year old

15

Opportunity and fulfilment

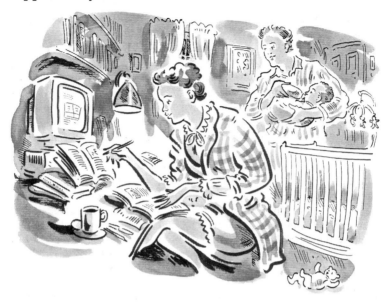

women benefit from relatively greater maturity and, perhaps, from a more highly developed social conscience.

Some ethnic minority groups, in particular those of South East Asian origin, apply for medicine (and for science and engineering) in far greater proportion than their number in the community. School-leavers of Afro-Caribbean origin, however, apply in relatively small numbers for reasons which have never been fully determined, but seem to include relatively low achievements at school. Medical schools would welcome an increased application from suitably qualified Afro-Caribbean applicants. The high application rate of Asians for medicine may arise from a keen personal scientific and humanitarian interest, from parental socioeconomic aspirations for their children, or from cultural tradition— or from a mixture of each.

Mature applicants have both advantages and disadvantages as medical students. Their experience of life, achievement, compassion for and contribution to others, and their commitment to a change of career for very positive, humanitarian, or, occasionally, scientific reasons is often most impressive. They contribute greatly to the stability and responsibility of their immediate year and more widely in the medical school as a whole, and their maturity is an advantage in communicating and empathising with patients. Applicants over the age of about 30 present medical schools with a difficult choice because admitting such a mature student excludes a younger person likely to work as a doctor for up to a decade longer.

Financial problems (and adjusting to them, having previously been self supporting) are their greatest handicap. Mature students are more likely to drop out from the medical course for financial than academic reasons, although some do find the return to academic work more difficult than anticipated. Mature students over the age of 25 are considered to be independent of their parents. If not previously in receipt of a grant for higher education they receive a mandatory grant for the whole course, means-tested on their own income. If they have already had a local education authority (LEA) grant they are most unlikely to get a discretionary grant for the pre-clinical course but they may be awarded a grant for two or three of the clinical years according to the policy (and means) of the LEA. The system is chancy and inequitable. Some medical schools, including my own, concentrate their scholarship resources on mature students because theirs is the greatest need, with both financial position and all-round achievement being taken into account. Details of any scholarships and how to enter for them can usually be found in a medical school's prospectus.

Apart from the financial difficulties which arise from different grant status and parental means or commitment, inequalities show at medical school in several other ways. Women, equal in number, at least equal in ability, and, by and large, more mature, live happily and achieve excellently in a community which has residually and perhaps curiously a somewhat "macho" male dominated ethos. A handful of teachers steeped in this tradition may still appear condescending or even dismissive towards women (and towards black students) but their outdated attitude is more likely to be directed towards students in general rather than women or any other subset of students in particular. Maturer students are understandably particularly sensitive to and outraged by such attitudes. Patients are generally as happy with women as with men but some may still be unfriendly to students from ethnic minorities.

A small but significant minority of Asian women students are subject to family pressures which are sufficient to destroy their ability to cope happily or effectively with their work. Parents and grandparents may limit their freedom, demand their frequent presence (a demand not limited to the women students or indeed to Asian families), and even force them into arranged marriages. Deans are familiar with situations in which they have to send down students for academic failure due to such pressures. It may be necessary to tell parents in such circumstances that until they are prepared to give their children personal and intellectual liberty these students cannot be readmitted because effective work under the strain of such a culture clash has proved impossible. Families of any section of the student population may of course make

demands difficult to reconcile with the student's effective performance, deliberately or inadvertently, reasonably or unreasonably.

Mature students, especially those with families to care for and
support, face the most predictable conflicts between their studies
and other responsibilities. The early years, with standard university terms and no essential out of hours commitments, are no more
difficult for medicine than other degree courses, except to the
extent that the intensity of lectures and practical work is greater
than for most other subjects. Efficient use of time during the day
and a regular hour or two of study most evenings (and more before
examinations) should suffice. Some students manage to support
themselves by evening and weekend jobs at this stage but it is not
easy; and during the clinical course it is more or less impossible
and certainly most undesirable. The clinical years are each 48
weeks long with holidays normally at set times. Most of the clinical
assignments require one night or weekend in hospital every week
or two. Two or three "residencies"—for example, in obstetrics or
paediatrics—require living in a distant hospital for a week or two at
a time, taking every possible opportunity to learn from the work in
progress, including, within limits, at night. Apart from this, the
clinical student's day is likely to start at 0800 or 0900 hours and
finish at about 1700 hours with weekends free. The elective period
of two to three months is often spent abroad but assignments may
be arranged close to home which will not necessarily involve night
or weekend duty.

Good organisation, a sufficient income, and an understanding
partner with a flexible job are the foundations from which medicine may successfully be studied by women with children. One
such student started just over the age of 30 with two children aged
between 5 and 10 and a husband willing and able to adjust his
working hours to hers. The higher education college at which she
was studying for A levels described her as the most outstanding
student, academically and personally, that they could remember.
She won several prizes on her way through the course and
qualified without difficulty. Another of similar age with four
children and separated from her husband coped with such amazing
energy and effectiveness despite considerable financial hardship
(and the help of a succession of au-pairs) that she left everyone
breathless. Exceptional she may be but it can be done, requiring as
Susan Spindler commented in her book *Doctors To Be*, ".. an
unerring sense of priorities in her life, tremendous stamina and the
capacity to concentrate briefly but hard."

Requirements for entry

It is as possible for a man to know something without having been to school as it is to have been to school and know nothing.

HENRY FIELDING *Tom Jones*

The A level requirements select people too academic for a career which needs compassion, endurance, and a damn good memory, rather than brains.

R JOHNSTON (1981)

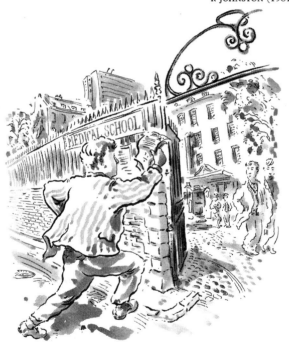

The academic standard of most applicants to universities in England, Wales and Northern Ireland has until now been judged largely on their performance in the General Certificate of Education (GCE) at advanced (A) level. A good grade in chemistry or physical science at A level, or in chemistry at AS level, is required by all universities. Most universities will also consider admission on the strength of results in the full international baccalaureate including chemistry and in the Scottish Certificate of Education

Requirements for entry

(SCE). Chemistry in the European baccalaureate has generally not been an acceptable substitute for A level but several universities now accept it; its position in relation to an AS requirement has yet to be established. Alternatively an honours degree of first or upper second class may be accepted. Otherwise the candidate will have to pass a 1st MB examination (see below).

Most Scottish applicants to Scottish medical schools and a few who apply outside Scotland are admitted on their results in the Scottish certificate; they are also generally required to study for an additional year after taking the SCE and to pass the Scottish Certificate of Sixth Year Studies, taken at the end of that year.

Applicants offering the Scottish Certificate outside Scotland should clarify their position with the universities of their choice before completing their UCAS (Universities and Colleges Admissions Service) applications. London University, for example, requires a good grade in the Certificate of Sixth Year Studies as well as the SCE.

With entrance on GCE A level achievement, universities usually require two other science subjects at GCE A level taken from the group of physics (unless physical science is offered), biology, and mathematics. Sometimes a good grade in an arts subject may be accepted in place of one (and occasionally two) other science subjects.

All universities will accept a combination of A levels and AS levels (see table I). Universities differ in the subjects which may be offered at AS level: London University, for example, requires that one at least must be in a maths or a science subject not being offered at A level. For entry to the premedical year where that is offered, two AS levels can always be substituted for one A level. Those offering arts subjects are required to have good passes in the General Certificate of Secondary Education (GCSE) in the sciences or mathematics not offered. Special arrangements may be made for mature students who are not university graduates, but they are unlikely to be excused the requirement for chemistry.

Universities do not generally express a preference between A level mathematics and biology for medicine. More applicants still offer biology but about 40% offer mathematics instead. Chemistry and biology are the foundations of basic medical science, especially if the mathematical aspects of those subjects are included. However useful it may be to be numerate in medicine, especially in research, students without a good knowledge of biology find themselves handicapped, at least in the first year, by their lack of understanding of cell and organ function and its terminology. They also generally have greater difficulty in expressing themselves in writing, especially if their first language is not English.

Requirements for entry

TABLE I—Most flexible A level combination acceptable and typical grades required at first attempt for entry to medicine (excluding premedical, 1st MB, courses)

Medical school	Typical A level grades required	Chemistry* + 2 science or maths	Chemistry* + 1 science or maths	Chemistry* + 2 other
University of Birmingham	ABB		√	
University of Bristol	BBB		√	
University of Cambridge	AAA	√		
University of Leeds	ABB			√
University of Leicester	BBB	√		
University of Liverpool	ABB		√	
University of London:				
Charing Cross and Westminster	BBC		√	
King's	BBB		√	
The Royal London	BBB		√	
Royal Free	BBB		√	
St Bartholomew's	BBB		√	
St George's	BBC			√
Imperial College (St Mary's)	BBB			√
United Schools of Guy's and St Thomas's	BBC		√	
University College	BBB			√
University of Manchester	BBB			√
University of Newcastle upon Tyne	ABB			√
University of Nottingham	ABB			√
University of Oxford	AAA/AAB		√	
University of Sheffield	ABB		√	
University of Southampton	BBB			√
Queens University, Belfast	ABB	√		
University of Aberdeen	ABB	√		
University of Dundee	BBC	√		
University of Edinburgh	ABB		√	
University of Glasgow	BBB	√		
University of St Andrews	ABB		√	
University of Wales	ABB		√	

Notes: Requirements of schools are likely to change and should always be confirmed before application. The information is based on *University and College Entrance: Official Guide 1994*.

*Two AS levels may be substituted for one (and only one) A level including chemistry (see p 20).

Failure in the first two years of the course is commoner in those who did not take biology at A level.

The increased popularity of mathematics relative to biology is not so much because of changed perceptions of the value of mathematics for medicine but partly a function of its general usefulness for entry to alternative science courses and partly because good mathematicians (or average mathematicians with

Requirements for entry

good teachers?) can expect better grades in mathematics than in the more descriptive subject of biology.

All universities require good grades in biology, physics, and mathematics in GCSE if not offered at A level (see table I) together with English language. An increasing number of universities now accept integrated or combined science in GCSE. Oxford and Cambridge require another language besides English. A few applicants gain excellent grades at A level in four subjects—chemistry, physics, biology, and mathematics, or the less appropriate combination for medicine of chemistry, physics or biology, mathematics, and higher mathematics. It is a better strategy for admission to achieve three good grades than four indifferent ones.

Different but equally rigorous academic achievement may be accepted in the case of mature students, including graduates.

ARTS SUBJECTS

Far from one or even two arts subjects being a second best (provided the GCSE grades in science and mathematics are excellent) much can be said in favour of languages, literature, and history as a path to greater sensitivity, insight, and human understanding. Some applicants have already acquired maturity of personality through their own experience in turbulent homes or difficult schools, in spare time activities directed towards the needs of others, or in earning their own living, but most know little of the world at large and are very limited in the breadth of their intellectual development. Not many applicants take advantage of the option of offering non-science subjects at A level for entry to medicine. At some schools the problem is of timetabling a mixture of arts and science. Other schools seem not to believe that the option to combine arts and science is taken seriously by medical schools. In fact the success rate in application and the grades achieved by those offering some arts subjects is similar to those offering only science subjects.

Those who have had an inadequate background of science at school must either study science at A level at a college of further education or take a premedical 1st MB course. With determination, application, and talent applicants lacking school science can study successfully part time for science A level examinations while continuing to earn their living, an achievement which is an impressive recommendation for acceptance into medicine. Only seven universities still offer a 1st MB course (see table II) and these courses are no longer designed for students with poor A level science but for non-scientists with a good academic record in their own subjects. A 1st MB course lasts one year and, contrary to information in earlier editions of this book, a

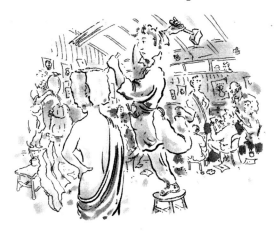

medical course that includes a 1st MB year does qualify for a mandatory local education authority grant.

Students who, commendably, have wider academic interests than their science A level subjects are often uncertain whether to offer an extra subject such as music or art at A level. Such a heavy undertaking may be a risk in so far as it may jeopardise the grades obtained in the main subjects, but a very different subject may on the other hand act more as relaxation than harmful diversion. Nevertheless, it may be wiser not to study it as part of an examination programme. Applicants do sometimes regret their temerity, such as the boy who wrote an apology for his science A level grades, which were less good than expected though complemented by a grade B in sculpture:

> My own feeling is that a partial cause of my poor performance was my failure to abandon A level sculpture after the papers had arrived two weeks late (they had been lost in the post), which caused a clash between the time consuming process of casting and preparation for life drawing and my peak revision period. . . . In retrospect, it is little consolation both to have finished and perhaps even won the game of bowls but to have been defeated by the Armada.

Since the circumstances under which applicants study for A level vary and since schools differ greatly in the quality of their facilities and teaching some flexibility over entry requirements is called for. Targets and especially achievements need to be balanced with a realism based on opportunity; the search should above all be for potential, and targets occasionally need to be tailored to candidates of good potential but poor opportunity. In practice it is simpler to identify schools and tutorial colleges which are efficient examination result factories than it is to know which schools are under-privileged in staff or environment.

Requirements for entry

If it is correct to conclude that, apart from chemistry and possibly biology, advanced studies at school are largely for intellectual development rather than for their factual content in relation to a subsequent medical education, it follows that the choice of subjects offered is not critical and that grades are primarily important as a reasonable surety that the medical course will not present insuperable academic difficulty. Under average circumstances of study this "surety" level of minimum achievement in science subjects seems to be not lower than grade C at the first attempt after two years of study, although many schools demand a minimum of B at first attempt because of intense competition. The fact that mean A level achievements in many subjects have risen recently without any convincing evidence that applicants to university are academically more able is tending to force upwards the "surety" level. For this reason, and in the pressure of competition, many medical schools are poised to raise their minimum requirements. It is difficult to estimate scientific ability from arts results (even assuming excellent O level science), and higher grades may be expected in arts than in science if only to counter criticisms of an easy backdoor entry to medicine.

FAILING FIRST TIME ROUND

What then of those who take longer before a first attempt or retake the examinations after further study? Clearly there are perfectly acceptable reasons for poor performance at first attempt, such as illness, bereavement, and multiple change of school. One unusual reason, perhaps indicating an inquiring if somewhat incompetent mind, was pleaded by a headmaster who explained that a candidate's "illegitimate chemical experiments cost him a large part of the summer term." Under these circumstances the best course is for the student to resit the examination, within months if possible (which it is with some examination boards and not with others) and to hope that the original grade targets will stand. If it is necessary to wait a year a higher target is usually set. A second conditional offer is by no means automatic because competition is new each year.

Three points might be made about applicants who for no good reason perform below target at first attempt. Firstly, a modest polishing of grades confers little additional useful knowledge and gives no promise of improved potential for further development, especially when only one or two subjects are retaken; the less there is to do the better it should be done, and the medical course itself requires the ability to keep several subjects on the boil simultaneously. On the other hand, a dramatic improvement (unless achieved by highly professional "cramming") may indicate late development or reveal desirable and necessary qualities of determination and application. Secondly, age too must be taken into account. The usual age for taking A level is 18 and younger applicants may simply have been taken through school too fast. Thirdly, the failure rate in the first two years of the course is higher among those who failed to achieve their A level grades at first attempt.

GRADES

The minimum grades expected for admission (grades range from A to E) differ from school to school (see table I), although the grades actually achieved by entrants vary much less. My school previously set a modest target of B in chemistry with two C grades, but 27% of entrants achieved AAA in 1993 and 86% achieved BBB or better. Very few people are admitted to medicine with three C grades and if there is no reasonable prospect of doing better than that at first attempt it is generally wiser to consider an alternative course.

Far more applicants could cope academically with the course in medicine than can be accepted. Some schools select more or less entirely on the basis of high grades; others set a more modest target but put more emphasis on less measurable qualities such as commitment, perseverance, determination, initiative, originality, and concern for others. These qualities are judged from the UCAS application form and from interview. Opinion is widely split on the value of interview in selection, but, whatever its shortcomings, most medical schools interview all their most promising applicants and no school never interviews at all.

Personality, attitude, and the ability to communicate do not figure on the list of minimum requirements, but there is no doubt that these attributes matter. It is, however, easier to judge, from a combination of confidential report and interview, the few relatively unsuitable than between the many who would be suitable. Occupations within medicine are admittedly very diverse, but most medical posts require the ability to communicate with and to care for people and the training itself certainly requires the ability to communicate. Medicine is a university degree course but it is not confined to theoretical study and laboratory benchwork; in the clinical years (apart from the pathology teaching) hospital wards and clinics and general practitioners' surgeries and patients' homes are the laboratories and patients are the reagents. Students who do not relate well to patients may certainly have a contribution to make to medical science, but their best route, at least so far as the patients themselves are concerned, may well be through a science and not a medical degree.

Choosing a medical school

A few boys are incorrigibly idle, and a few are incorrigibly eager for knowledge; but the great mass are in a state of doubt and fluctuation, and they come to school for the express purpose, not of being left to themselves—for that could be done anywhere—but that their wavering tastes and propensities should be decided by the intervention of a master.

SYDNEY SMITH (nineteenth century)

Through all the variations it may be possible to identify four major themes responsible for the excellence one senses in teaching the art of medicine:
(1) selection of bright students responsive to the excitement of both science and the care of patients
(2) selection or recruitment of bright teachers who are anxious to remain students all their lives and who also derive joy from teaching
(3) an atmosphere of discovery—an ever expanding search for truth and correction of error, no matter whose
(4) facilities and support making it possible for bright students to learn and the bright teachers to teach as they continue to learn.

SHERMAN M MELLINKOFF (1987)

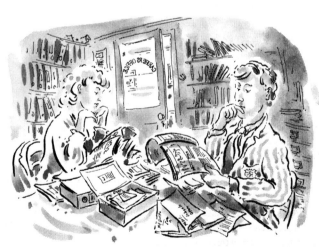

Choice of career is one of the most far reaching decisions of your life. Having decided, realistically, to learn medicine, the next question is—where? The outcome of that choice has profound academic, professional, and, in all probability, personal consequences.

TABLE II—*Entry of UK students to basic medical science courses in United Kingdom medical schools in 1993*

Medical school	Entry	Applications per place
University of Birmingham	163	11
University of Bristol*	133	12
University of Cambridge	200	4
University of Leeds†	208	13
University of Leicester	139	12
University of Liverpool	184	9
University of London		
Charing Cross and Westminster	151	10
King's	117	15
The Royal London	87	16
Royal Free	96	17
St Bartholomew's	109	8
St George's	186	9
Imperial College (St Mary's)	115	20
United Schools of Guy's and St Thomas's	210	7
University College	174	19
University of Manchester*	238	12
University of Newcastle upon Tyne*	151	11
University of Nottingham	138	19
University of Oxford	96	6
University of Sheffield*	123	12
University of Southampton	154	11
Queen's University, Belfast	155	5
University of Aberdeen	147	7
University of Dundee*	128	12
University of Edinburgh*	174	11
University of Glasgow	226	6
University of St Andrews	81	7
University of Wales*	178	8

*Application and acceptance figures include premedical (1st MB) course.
†Application and acceptance figures include non-clinical three year medical sciences courses.
Note: The number of overseas students permitted at medical schools in the UK is approximately 7·5% of total intake.

The environment of learning fashions intellectual development, attitudes, and horizons; it also adds the finishing touches to personality. More likely than not, the site where student days are spent also determines life's partner. Some of the particular academic and personal influences exerted by a university can be predicted from its courses, traditions, and location. Much is as unpredictable as the pattern of coloured pieces in a kaleidoscope of students given an annual shake for each university, college, and course.

No such momentous decision is normally taken on such scanty information. Prospectuses often fail to answer the important questions; medical advisers are usually fiercely loyal to their old school but wildly out of date; and careers teachers usually do not succeed in keeping up with change or in fully assessing the effects of change on students. Today's students are the best guides to tomorrow's on the atmosphere of a school and on the acceptability

Choosing a medical school

of its course, if not its academic merits—which they may not perceive so clearly (though they know what they like). Personal inclination apart, is the aspiration to go to a particular university medical school realistic in the light of personal qualifications and competition from others?

ACADEMIC CONSIDERATIONS

The 28 university medical schools in the UK, of which nine are in London, vary considerably in size (see table II), atmosphere, environment, and emphasis of their courses. All these university medical schools turn out capable doctors and if you really want to learn medicine you should be prepared to go wherever an opportunity exists. But your pleasure in the process and your horizons on qualification depend very much on matching your personality to that of your medical school. The most important outcome of differences in approach is not professional competence but inspiration. Inspiration arises partly from a predictable interplay between the type of course and personal interests, and partly from a more chancy striking of sparks on the one hand between imaginative teachers and responsive students and on the other between fellow students.

Three major differences of approach can be discerned, but their edges are blurred. A few universities, of which Oxford and Cambridge are the prime, study in depth the sciences particularly related to medicine (anatomy, physiology, biochemistry, pharmacology, and pathology) as disciplines important in their own right, primarily as tools of intellectual development and scientific education rather than of vocational equipment; clinical relevance does not receive great emphasis.

The Oxford and Cambridge preclinical courses take three years and lead to a bachelor of arts degree, notwithstanding the scientific nature of the course. Each has its considerable merits.

At Oxford all the anatomy, physiology, biochemistry, and pharmacology required for the professional qualifications are covered in the first, intensive five terms' work and are then examined in the first BM. All students then take in their remaining four terms the honours school in physiology, a wider course than its name suggests, with options to choose from in the subjects of physiology, anatomy, biochemistry, pathology, and experimental psychology.

Cambridge adopts a more flexible approach. All the essential components of the course are covered in two years. The last year is spent studying in depth one of a number of subjects, the choice being determined partly by whether or not the student is going on to take the conventional London or Oxford clinical course or the shorter Cambridge clinical course. For students taking the Cambridge clinical course choice is limited to subjects approved by the General Medical Council as "a year of medical study": apart from the normal preclinical subjects these include subjects such as physical anthropology, social and political sciences, and zoology. Those taking a conventional clinical course subsequently at London or another university have the attractive opportunity to spend their third preclinical year reading for a part II in any subject—law, music, or whatever takes their fancy—provided they have a suitable educational background and their local education authority is sufficiently inspired to support them. A new option at Cambridge offers a few selected students the opportunity to combine study for a PhD with a modified clinical course.

The Oxford and Cambridge preclinical courses are the strongest on science, provide the greatest purely intellectual stimulation, and are most likely to awake academic interest and to broaden academic horizons. They are, however, less directly concerned than most other courses with the applications of science in medicine and they give more emphasis to traditional biological sciences and less to the newer, "softer," behavioural sciences (psychology and sociology). St Andrews, the only university with a preclinical course and no clinical school, also has a separate three year preclinical course which leads to the degree of BSc (medical science).

Nottingham is the only other university to award a science degree routinely to all successful students after three years, in their case a bachelor of medical science (BMedSci). The structure of the curriculum is, however, quite different in that it combines basic medical sciences and relevant aspects of clinical medicine from the beginning.

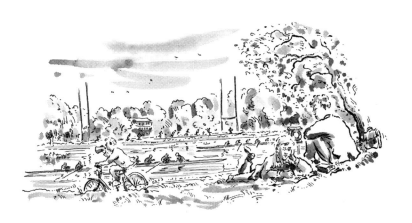

Choosing a medical school

Students at other medical schools have the opportunity to take an "intercalated" BSc (or at Newcastle BMedSci) in an additional year normally intercalated between the second pre-clinical year and the beginning of the clinical course. In addition to the conventional intercalated degree, a BSc course in clinical science, which is normally taken between the second and final clinical years, is offered in London University (see p 54).

For students of most medical schools which do not offer an honours degree in science as a standard part of the course, the BSc or BMedSci provides their best opportunity to explore, discover, and consider. It also provides a first step in developing skills in medical research. Southampton gives all students a project combining clinical and basic medical sciences which occupies most of the fourth year but this does not lead to a science degree.

In choosing a medical school it is important to note that in addition to whether or not they lead to a science degree, preclinical courses differ both in their "horizontal" integration, the extent to which they teach about body systems rather than separate departmental subjects, and in their "vertical" integration, the mixing of clinical medicine with basic medical science.

Multidisciplinary teaching directed towards body systems has the advantage of minimising repetition and of harmonising the different aspects of a particular topic. At the same time interdepartmental teaching is more difficult to organise and is in some respects more time consuming and difficult to examine satisfactorily. The degree of interdepartmental teaching matters less to the students than the quality of teaching itself, but they nevertheless usually welcome attempts by teachers to coordinate and combine their teaching.

Most medical schools are in the process of planning and introducing curricula which better integrate knowledge of medical science (including behavioural science) with its clinical applications, often by centering the teaching in the early years of the course around clinical problems. The factual load is being reduced and a core course with a series of options for study in more depth is being devised. Much greater emphasis will be given in future to self directed learning, communication skills, and decision-making.

Students like to have some clinical insights during the preclinical course. Most schools use patients in clinical demonstrations to illustrate normal mechanisms through the consequences of their failure. Many also attach a student to a family chosen by a local general practitioner at the beginning of the course to provide insight and human interest from the outset. Several schools give some instruction in clinical methods in the second preclinical year but few would claim that the amount of instruction given at that stage does more than arouse interest, strengthen motivation, and encourage a continued awareness of the human interrelationships and communication on which good medical care depends.

The exception is Nottingham, where students start talking and listening to patients and examining them in the first year and continue with an increasing clinical involvement throughout the course. Many students elsewhere are quite content or even prefer to concentrate first on the scientific basis of medicine and human behaviour and to defer personal contact with patients until they are older, perhaps wiser, and able to give themselves wholly to the task of developing clinical skills.

The clinical course at all universities lasts two years and nine months, except at Cambridge and Nottingham, where it lasts two years and three months. Most of the clinical course is a matter of listening and talking to patients and examining them under supervision; at most schools lectures play a small part. Students learn better when given opportunities to participate in decisions of diagnosis and management, made to feel useful, and encouraged to take responsibility. A Chinese proverb puts the philosophy in a nutshell: "I hear and I forget; I see and I remember; I do and I understand."

Applicants to medical school have little chance of making a realistic appraisal of various clinical courses as clinical education is even further removed from their own experience than the pre-clinical course. It is, however, clearly difficult to feel involved and to learn at the back of a large group gathered around a patient's bed, so one thing to look for is the size of the clinical "firms" (see p 59), a group of five or six students being the optimum in most circumstances. Emphasis given in the prospectus to students taking responsibility is another good sign. A balance of teaching between the rather specialised main university hospital and other more everyday district general hospitals is appropriate, but best when most of the experience outside the main teaching hospital is undertaken near enough to base for students to continue to follow a core course of lectures and topic teaching on one day a week and to continue to participate in the life of the school.

Experience of the provision and organisation of medical care outside hospital is an important and increasingly popular aspect of clinical training, which is provided both in general practice and in public health attachments. It is worth noting how much emphasis is given to these subjects. The prospectus will usually answer the question but you may need to ask at interview.

LIFE OF THE UNIVERSITY AND MEDICAL SCHOOL

The life and spirit of your place of study for five or six years could well be a more important weight in the balance of choice of

Choosing a medical school

medical school than differences in the detail of the course itself. The course is long, the amount of information to be learnt large, and encounter with patients emotionally demanding. Most medical schools are situated in rather grim parts of large cities, which is ideal for learning but often hard for living. Students are encouraged and supported through their training both by each other and by staff. The life of the medical school and university becomes their anchor and refreshment. Good relationships between students themselves and between staff and students make for teamwork which lifts an institution far above the demands of daily work and provides an inspiring sense of identity, common purpose, and enthusiasm.

The situation of medical students within different universities falls broadly into three groups. Oxford and Cambridge offer the attractions of multidisciplinary college life, an immense range of cultural and sporting activities within college and university, and a tutorial system which provides very personal direction of a student's work. Yet not everyone warms to the cloistered, still rather aristocratic abstraction of Oxbridge.

Provincial medical schools also offer a multidisciplinary setting to medical student life but without the distinctive Oxbridge college system. As medical students have a way of aggregating like crystals, keeping their own company and generating their own social life, they may often not benefit as much as might be supposed from the multidisciplinary but diffuse non-collegiate life of provincial universities. Moreover, these universities tend to have a large local element to their student body with a tradition of living at home or of returning home at weekends rather to the disadvantage of university life.

The faculty of medicine of London University is scattered in a mixture of multifaculty colleges and of solely medical (and some-times dental) colleges. Most of the main teaching hospitals and medical schools are older than the university itself. King's College Hospital Medical School, St Mary's Hospital Medical School, and University College Medical School are all part of multifaculty colleges, St Mary's being part of Imperial College of Science, Technology, and Medicine. Queen Mary College in the east end of London (not to be confused with St Mary's Hospital Medical School at Paddington in west London) has become part of a federation with The London Hospital Medical College and St Bartholomew's Hospital Medical College, the preclinical teaching being centred on the Queen Mary College site. St Mary's Hospital Medical School continues to be integrated with St Mary's Hospital in Paddington and to preserve its own distinct personality and name while at the same time benefiting from and contributing to the larger educational, scientific, and social framework of the

Imperial College campus straddling Hyde Park and Kensington Gardens.

The remaining medical schools within the faculty of medicine of London University are solely medical (or medical and dental), attached to a university hospital on the same site. While their situation might breed narrow medical isolation, removed from the formative cultural and sporting activities of a university, the truth is the reverse. Many of these students live for part of their course in general London University halls of residence which accept students from all colleges and faculties. Wherever they live or study, medical students share as fully as any others in the sporting and cultural life of the university as a whole. College life in London University tends to be more active than university life: London medical schools have a long tradition of accepting academically able students on the basis of their wider interests, abilities, and attitudes, not on A level grades alone. This policy makes for a widely talented active student society, most active in general at schools well endowed with their own local accommodation—a point worth looking for in the prospectus. In sport, music, and drama some individual medical schools could hold their own with many a whole university. Spirit and wide talent, together with the close staff–student relationships possible in a small institution, more than compensate for relative isolation within the university.

As a result of the Tomlinson Report into the arrangement of teaching hospitals and medical schools in London, it is likely that the United Medical School of Guy's and St Thomas's will become part of King's College; that the Royal London and St Bartholomew's Medical Colleges will merge with each other and with Queen Mary Westfield College; that the Royal Free Hospital Medical School will merge with University College Medical School; and it is possible that Charing Cross and Westminster Medical School will merge into Imperial College (forming with the existing Medical School of Imperial, St Mary's, a new Imperial College School of Medicine). All these changes will take time, if they happen at all, and are not likely adversely to affect the lives or education of students entering in 1995.

TRANSFER TO MEDICINE AND BETWEEN MEDICAL SCHOOLS

The intake of medical students in the UK is tightly controlled by the Higher Education Funding Council on the direction of the Department of Health, which is responsible for forecasting the number of doctors the country needs or, more accurately, is prepared to pay for.

Medical schools do not normally consider students who wish to transfer to medicine internally or from another university. It is not worth those who applied unsuccessfully for medicine and are now taking an alternative course to attempt to transfer at this stage. An occasional highly able student who never applied for medicine but now has had a change of heart is sometimes lucky. In general, however, deans take the attitude that a student who has begun another university degree course should finish and do well in that before being eligible for consideration for medicine. From the student's point of view the disadvantage in waiting is that a local education authority will transfer and continue a mandatory grant to a new course after one year but not at a later stage; some authorities are prepared to give graduates in other subjects a discretionary grant for two or three clinical years.

About 120 Oxbridge graduates undertake clinical studies at London University medical schools, thus achieving a nice balance of experience between dreaming spires and teeming streets. Some Cambridge graduates go to Oxford for clinical studies, a few go from Oxford to Cambridge and a handful of London intercalated BSc graduates undertake their clinical studies at either Oxford or Cambridge. These pathways of interchange are well worn and are now embraced in one simple common application procedure. A handful of Oxbridge graduates take their clinical studies at provincial universities and an occasional student moves in the opposite direction.

Apart from the Oxbridge-centred interchanges, transfers between medical schools are difficult to achieve because of different course timings and specific university regulations. Students who wish to transfer to another university for their clinical course have to satisfy the university that their preclinical course has been equivalent in all substantial respects. Transfers between universities are not possible during the preclinical course and are generally only considered for the clinical course (other than the Oxbridge schemes) on compassionate grounds.

Preclinical, 1st MB, courses are an exception. The seven universities which offer premedical courses normally expect to take successful students into their own medical course but they do not stand in the way of students applying for good reasons to undertake their medical studies elsewhere. In this case, the student has to apply again through UCAS. Successful completion of a 1st MB course at one university makes an applicant eligible for admission to any other UK university but does not guarantee that the application will succeed.

LOCATION

The location of a medical school determines the emphasis of clinical experience and the detail of day to day experience of life.

The complex interrelationships between social, economic, and medical conditions cannot be escaped in the "cold, grey, grittiness" of the inner city. Large centres also attract many of the most difficult clinical cases and while these cases are far more important to postgraduate education and research than to undergraduates, the challenge of the frontiers of medicine attracts good clinical scientists and teachers. The widest experience of everyday disease relatively uncomplicated by social pressures is to be found in the country towns and city suburbs, and medical schools located in inner cities send their students out to balance and increase their experience.

About half the graduates of a medical school are said to end up practising within 50 miles of it. That being so, applicants intent on a lifetime in Northumbria would be wise to choose Newcastle University in preference to Bristol or Aberdeen. It is a sad fact that awareness of a north–south divide is one reason why applicants are reluctant to move far from home. Interchange is invigorating and should be encouraged; traditions are different but are readily harmonised with goodwill and a sense of humour.

Scotland and Northern Ireland may seem far away to most people in our bottom-heavy United Kingdom, but the universities of Scotland and Northern Ireland are relatively generously provided with medical student places. The fact that they currently accept mostly Scots and Irish, respectively, may reflect only the pattern of applications. It would be shortsighted to overlook the opportunities their universities offer to applicants from elsewhere in the UK.

Much can be said for studying away from the parental home, notwithstanding the national economic pressures which would force students to commute from home wherever possible. The life of the medical school, university, and hospital are an integral part of the process of medical education; this life is to be immersed in, not taken in measured doses. That is not to say that convenience does not enter somewhere into the equation, as with the Welsh students who for generations have ended up at the end of the South Wales to London railway line at St Mary's Hospital Medical School beside Paddington Station, or the young lady who told the dean of St George's Hospital Medical School, when it was at Hyde Park Corner, that she had applied there because it was on her way to Harrods.

SPECIFIC REQUIREMENTS

Having selected the medical schools at which you would most like to study it is essential to double check your qualifications or

Choosing a medical school

expected qualifications against their specific requirements. Many choices are wasted unnecessarily because applicants have not done this homework. This book cannot give a complete catalogue of the small print differences in the requirements of different universities or schools of one university. That is not in any case its purpose. Its purpose is to indicate what to look for and to persuade you to think and research for yourself. With a lifetime at stake a little time and trouble now can reasonably be expected and certainly will be repaid.

At the simplest level, there is no point in applying with less than an upper second in a previous degree or with A level grades which do not at least fulfil (or are expected to fulfil) the minimum requirements of your chosen schools, unless you have already made or will make a convincing case about mitigating circumstances. Note that if a school specifies a particular grade in a particular subject, usually chemistry or physical science, you must have it and cannot presume that averaging of grades across all your subjects will make up a deficiency. The pressure for places is such and the reasons for specifying particular grades, especially in chemistry, are so strongly argued that most medical schools do not average results.

It is not sensible to apply on the basis of a second attempt at A level to schools which say that they do not consider retake applicants unless there were special circumstances adversely affecting the performance at first attempt, unless of course you can make such a case. If you can, then by all means do. Arts subjects should not be wasted on universities which insist on all science or maths for medicine; if the prospectus is not clear about arts subjects, inquire about your own particular position before applying. There is no substitute for careful preparation of the ground: hope may spring eternal but hope alone opens few doors to medical school. Medical schools are, however, rapidly becoming more liberal in their requirements.

It is important not to overlook the fact that university matriculation requirements (the general entry requirements of universities) vary and that individual faculties often require more than the general regulations in GCSE and at A level. Check whether the university requires a second language in addition to English language. Most medical faculties or schools require biology, physics, and maths in GCSE if not offered at A together with chemistry (or physical science), but not all insist on either or both biology and physics. Most medical schools accept both separate science subjects and combined science in GCSE. If offering the Scottish certificate or the baccalaureate make sure that it is acceptable to your chosen universities.

Consider the interview. If you doubt your ability to survive an interview or object on principle, whatever the principle, choose schools which do not routinely interview. On the other hand if you wish to show your face, argue your case, and demonstrate your commitment, carefully consider going for schools which do interview.

Age is another consideration. If unusually young, make sure that you do not fall below the minimum age limit. Most schools do not normally admit students under the age of 18 at entry or on 31 December of the year of entry. If old, take note that few universities admit medical students over the age of 25 and none normally admits over the age of 30. Search out the doves from the prospectuses; send an exploratory letter with a curriculum vitae to the deans of the schools which seem most open minded, ideally before application, and do not apply over the age of 30 unless you can make a convincing case that you are in one way or another deserving of special consideration.

It is difficult to say which schools are, year by year, most welcoming to mature students, but both Southampton and St Mary's (Imperial College) have traditionally been particularly sympathetic to them.

Women often wonder whether as women they stand a better chance of acceptance at one school rather than another. The answer is no. The proportions of men and women in the intake of any particular school vary according to the chances of selection and examination performance from year to year, but overall the proportions are much the same and reflect the pattern of applications. In 1993 52·1% of first year students and 50·2% of all applicants were women.

Medical schools must be listed in their UCAS number order. If you have a strong and defensible reason for a particular preference it would be helpful to admission officers if that were mentioned in the confidential reference. Otherwise there are good reasons for simply taking your chance with your chosen shortlist.

Most medical schools have open days or are prepared to show potential applicants around. If at all possible arrange to visit the universities which interest you most. In all your dealings with medical schools search out answers for yourself. It is hard to understand why some young adults (and even occasional mature students) about to launch themselves on their careers should have their questions asked for them by their parents. The first way to persuade a university that your decisions are your own is to speak for yourself.

Application and selection

Are the clearly specified and hence readily defensible criteria those most likely to yield a wise and cultivated doctor—a person capable of dealing with uncertainty, of compassionate understanding and wise judgement? Can an ideal physician be expected from an intellectual *forme fruste* who has spent his college years only learning the "right answers"?

STEWART G WOLFE (1978)

The value of the Physician is derived far more from what may be called his general qualities than from his special knowledge ... such qualities as good judgement, the ability to see a patient as a whole, the ability to see all aspects of a problem in the right perspective, and the ability to weigh up evidence are far more important than the detailed knowledge of some rare syndrome.

JOHN TODD (1978)

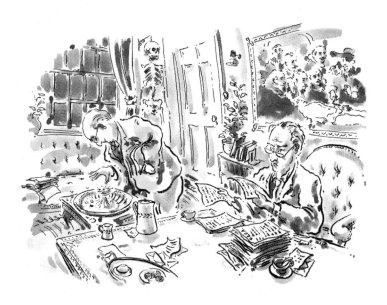

Unfortunately the qualities which count for most in medicine are not precisely measurable. The measurable—examination performance at school—neither necessarily relates to these qualities nor guarantees intellectual potential. Furthermore, there is no acceptable objective measure of the quality of a doctor against which to test the worth of earlier decisions. In this sea of uncertainty it is not surprising that selection processes are imperfect and open to criticism. Nonetheless few patients would choose a doctor without meeting him or her first, and a strong argument can be made for discovering the people behind their UCAS forms, if only briefly. Also, many applicants feel it only right that they should have an opportunity to put their own case.

Selection for interview (and at some schools for offer without interview) is made on the strength of an application submitted through UCAS, an application completed partly by the applicant and partly by a referee, usually the head or a member of the school staff, who submits a confidential reference.

Altogether about 10 800 home students and 1600 from overseas applied to read medicine in 1993; 4292 home students and 342 from overseas were accepted. Women comprised 50·2% of applicants and 52·1% of those accepted.

It is worth completing the UCAS form accurately and legibly. Deans and admissions tutors who have to scan a thousand or two application forms (which they receive reduced in size from the original application) simply do not have time to spend deciphering illegible handwriting. A legible, even stylish, presentation creates a good impression from the start.

PERSONAL DETAILS

The first section of the UCAS form presents the personal details of the applicant, including age on 30 September of the coming academic year. Many applicants give instead their current age and at a glance appear to fall below the minimum age for entry or to be so young that older applicants might reasonably be given priority over them. True, the date of birth is also requested, but the quickly scanning eye may not pick up the discrepancy.

The list of schools attended by an applicant is often a useful guide to the educational opportunity received. More ability and determination are needed to emerge as a serious candidate for medicine from a comprehensive school with 2000 pupils, of whom only 10–15 normally enter university each year, than from a selective school from which university entry is the norm. Multiple changes of school (usually because of parental mobility) are generally a disadvantage and need to be taken into account.

PREFERENCE

Fortunately, applicants are no longer expected to give all their course choices to medicine to indicate their strength of purpose.

Application and selection

Now that the eight universities or courses can be nominated on UCAS forms the medical schools have requested that applicants should limit the number of applications for medicine to five; an applicant unlikely to be successful with five choices is no more likely to succeed with eight. The remaining choices should be used for any alternative courses without prejudice to the applications for medicine.

The rumour that London University medical schools prefer to see all choices given to London is without foundation.

OTHER INFORMATION

Examination results should be clearly listed by year in the UCAS application form. It is sensible to list first those subjects immediately relevant to the science requirements for medicine and those subjects needed for university matriculation, usually English language, mathematics, and a foreign language. All attempts at examinations should be entered and clearly separated. The date and number of A level or degree examinations yet to be taken complete the picture.

While it probably never pays to try to amuse on an application form, it is worth being interesting. The section about interests, spare time activities, and practical experience presents an opportunity to catch the eye of a tired admissions dean, because medicine demands so much more than academic ability. Small details, such as the information that an applicant spends his free moments delivering newspapers, assisting in the village shop, and acting as "pall-bearer and coffin-carrier to the local undertaker" converts a cipher into a person. None of those particular activities should be immediately relevant to his future medical practice but at least they show initiative. Other activities, such as music, drama, and sport, indicate a willingness and ability to acquire practical skills and to participate, characteristics useful in life in general but also to a medical school, which needs its own cultural life to divert tired minds and to develop full personalities during a long course of training. Some applicants offer a remarkably wide variety of accomplishments, such as the boy who declared in his UCAS form:

> I play various types of music, including jazz, Irish traditional, orchestral and military band, on trombone, fiddle, tin whistle, mandolin and bohran. . . .

If Irish music be the food of medicine, play on. But that was not all, for he continued:

> I also enjoy boxing and I have a brown belt (Judo). My more sociable pastimes include ballroom dancing, photography, driving and motor cycling.

40

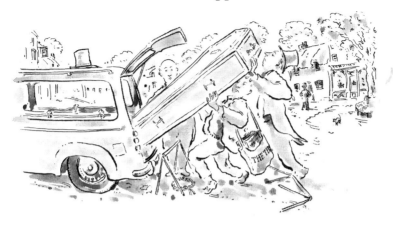

Would this young man have time for medicine?

It is not sensible to enter every peripheral interest and pastime lest it appears, as may indeed be so, that many of these activities are superficial. It is also unwise for an applicant to enter any interest that he or she would be unable to discuss intelligently at interview.

The applicant's own account of interests and the confidential report (for which a whole page is available) sometimes bring to life the different sides of an applicant's character. For example, one young man professed "a great interest in music" and confessed that he was "lead vocalist in a rowdy pop group" while his headmaster reported that he was "fairly quiet in lessons . . . science and medicine afford him good motivation . . . his choice of career suits him well. There is no doubt that he has the ability and temperament successfully to follow his calling." All in all this interplay of information is useful, for medicine is a suitable profession for multifaceted characters.

The confidential report is always important and is sometimes crucial. The headmaster, housemaster, or tutor usually takes great care to give a balanced, realistic assessment of progress and potential. Most teachers are painstaking over these confidential reports, and the few who are not (and they are very few) do their pupils a disservice. Readers of UCAS forms quickly discover the few schools pupilled entirely by angels. Cautionary nuances are more commonly conveyed by what is omitted than by what is said, but a few heads are sufficiently outspoken to write from the hip in appropriate circumstances. Frank but fair confidential references are an essential part of an acceptable selection process.

Application and selection

UCAS forms no longer include a formal prediction separate from the report itself of the grades expected at A level. Nevertheless, the confidential report usually includes a prediction of performance, which is more useful because it is set in the context of the report as a whole. Most schools manage to predict remarkably accurately and when wrong the fault is usually in overestimation. Occasionally a candidate is seriously underestimated, with the result that an interview is not offered and the applicant is at the mercy of the clearing procedure after the results are declared or has to apply again next year.

GETTING AN INTERVIEW

What in the mass of information counts in the decision to shortlist a candidate for interview or even, at some schools, for an offer without interview? I cannot speak for other schools but we pay attention especially to the grades achieved in GCSE and at A level if already taken; to outstanding achievement in any field, because excellence is not lightly achieved; to indications of determination, perseverance, and consideration for others; to an ability to communicate; to breadth and depth of other interests, especially to signs of originality; to the contribution likely to be made to the life of the school; to the confidential report; and to assessment of potential for further development taking all the evidence together. Highly though achievement is valued, potential, both personal and intellectual, is even more important. We look for applicants who are just beginning to get into their stride in preference to those who have already been forced to their peak, aptly described by Dorothy L Sayers in *Gaudy Night* as possessed of "small summery brains, that flower early and turn to seed."

Although our shortlisting process deliberately sets out to view applicants widely, analysis of the outcome has shown that academic achievement still carries the greatest weight in selecting candidates from their UCAS forms. The great majority of applicants called for interview are academically strong, and it is then that their personal characteristics decide the outcome (see next chapter).

Applicants could legitimately ask whether any factors, apart from the strength of the UCAS application form, enter into the selection for interview. It used to be customary at many medical schools (a tradition by no means confined to them) for the children of graduates of the school or of staff to be offered an interview, but that has now largely been abandoned out of conviction that the selection process must be, and be seen to be, open and, as far as can be, scrupulously fair.

Unsolicited letters of recommendation are a sensitive matter.

42

Application and selection

Factual information additional to the UCAS confidential report is occasionally important and is welcome from any source. For example, one applicant had left another medical school in his first term against the advice of his dean to work to support his mother and younger brother. Three years later, when the family was on its feet and he wanted to reapply to medical school, he was under a cloud for having given up his place. The UCAS form did not tell the full story, and a note from the family doctor was most helpful in giving the full background to a courageous and self sacrificing young man. Some other unsolicited letters add only the information that an applicant is either well connected or has good friends and it is difficult to see why such applicants should be given an advantage over those whose friends, weighty or not, do not feel it proper to canvass.

It is not only unsolicited testimonials that recommend in glowing terms. How could any dean resist the angel described thus by her headmaster:

> The charm of her personal character defies analysis. She is possessed of all the graces and her noble qualities impress everybody. She has proved the soul of courtesy and overlying all her virtues is sound common sense. She has always been mindful of her obligations and has fulfilled her responsibilities and duties as a prefect admirably well. Amiable and industrious, she appears to have a spirit incapable of boredom and her constructive loyalty to the school, along with her unfailing good nature, has won her the high esteem and admiration of staff and contemporaries alike.
> We recommend her warmly as a top drawer student.

A "top drawer" student indeed—and a top drawer headmaster.

WHEN TO APPLY

When is it best to apply: in September at the first opportunity, in October/November, or at the last possible moment? Apply as early as possible because applications reach schools from September to January and applicants are selected for interview or offer sequentially, as applications are received. Allowing for the fact that early applications are overall stronger than late ones, it is now clear that, all other things being equal, early applicants are more likely to receive an interview and therefore an offer, and by Christmas most of the offers a school can give have been given.

In principle a year's break between school and university is a good thing. The year is particularly valuable if used to experience the discipline and, often, the drudgery of earning a living from relatively unskilled work. It can provide insights for students (most of whom come from relatively well off families) into the everyday life and thinking of the community which will provide most of their patients in due course. There is no need for such work to be in the setting of health care; in fact much is to be said for escaping from the environment of doctors and hospitals.

If the earnings of these months (or the whole period on a Voluntary Service Overseas scheme) are then used to discover something of different cultures abroad that is a bonus. But just being a year older, more experienced, and more mature is helpful to the discipline and motivation of study and especially useful when faced with patients in the clinical course. In practice, short-term employment may, unfortunately, be difficult to find but there are few places where work of some description cannot be obtained if a student is prepared to do anything legal, however menial.

Settling down to academic work again after a year off can be a problem but it is not insuperable if the motivation and self discipline are there. If commitment has evaporated after a year's break, better to have discovered early than late; better to drop out before starting rather than to waste a place that another could use and to waste your own time which could better be channelled elsewhere.

A practical dilemma arises over whether to apply for deferred entry before taking A levels or early the year afterwards. Universities may be reluctant to commit themselves a year ahead to average applicants because the standard of applicants seems to be rising all the time. Outstanding applicants should, however, have no difficulty in arranging deferred entry before taking A level, but it is worth checking the policy of schools in which you are interested before applying. If not offered a deferred place, apply early the next year and send a covering letter to the deans of your chosen medical schools asking for as early an interview as possible if you are planning to go abroad.

Interviews and offers

The student who is not curious is surely no student at all; he is already old, and his thoughts are borrowed thoughts.

CHARLES WILSON (later Lord Moran) (1932)

Medicine is in some ways the most personal and responsible profession; the patient entrusts his life and well being to his doctor. Thus, the character and personality of the doctor, his sympathy and understanding, his sense of responsibility, his selflessness are as important as his scientific and technical knowledge.

SIR GEORGE PICKERING (1965)

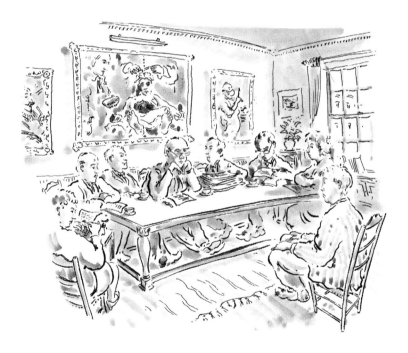

Opinion differs widely and deeply on the value and fairness of an interview as part of the process for selecting medical students. Two thirds of medical schools interview the strongest applicants and use the interview to decide between them; the remainder interview only a small number of applicants, such as mature students, in an

Interviews and offers

attempt to assess more fully their motivation and circumstances. Applicants who object to interviews, who doubt their ability to speak up for themselves, or who think that in speaking up they may prejudice their chances of admission can confine their applications to schools which normally do not interview (table III).

TABLE III—*Interviewing policies of United Kingdom medical schools according to whether or not they normally interview shortlisted applicants*

	Interviews		Interviews
Birmingham	Yes	United Schools of Guy's	
Bristol	Yes	and St Thomas's	Yes
Cambridge	Yes	Manchester	No
Leeds	Yes	Newcastle	Yes
Leicester	Yes	Nottingham	Yes
Liverpool	Yes	Oxford	Yes
London:		Sheffield	Yes
Charing Cross and		Southampton	No
Westminster	Yes	Belfast	No
King's	Yes	Aberdeen	No
The Royal London	Yes	Dundee	No
Royal Free	Yes	Edinburgh	No
St Bartholomew's	Yes	Glasgow	No
St George's	Yes	St Andrews	Yes
Imperial College (St Mary's)	Yes	Wales	Yes
University College	Yes		

If medicine were merely another university degree course selection would present fewer problems. As it is, learning medicine is a preparation for a professional career, a career which demands more than academic ability. So great are the uncertainties about who is most suitable for the task that some would argue for admission by a lottery governed by chance alone.

The purpose of an interview in my view is to explore whether individuals can communicate; can reason, not merely regurgitate knowledge; have made their own decisions rather than gravitating into a mould determined by parents or environment; and have some idea of the course and profession to which they aspire. The interview also provides an opportunity to visit a school, to meet staff and students, and to ask questions. Some schools achieve these ends by holding an open day. It is remarkably short sighted of an applicant to come to interview without having discovered as much about the school and its course as can be learnt from the prospectus, but, surprisingly, some do not take the trouble.

WEIGHING ACADEMIC AND OTHER FACTORS

The essence of arguments about interviews as a means of selection is whether or not the objective but possibly chancy, small, and, for the future, arbitrary difference of one grade should be given more weight than the subjective impression of personality and commitment. In this matter, as in so many others, there is no absolute truth. Fortunately admission policies differ, and candidates can choose the schools which adopt the approach they prefer.

The time and trouble involved in interviews are in my view justified by several considerations, especially by the opportunity they provide for applicants to speak for themselves. Interviews not only provide a method of choosing between a large number of people who seem equal on paper but also give a chance to those with less on paper because of special circumstances. Some of the latter make such a good impression at interview that they win an offer which would not have been forthcoming on their academic record alone. The challenge for the school is to call as many of these people to interview as possible, but they are hard to identify. By the same token a few who are brilliant on paper seem so lacking in either humanity, motivation, or personality that they lose at interview an offer which would otherwise have seemed a foregone conclusion. Most of those rejected after interview are not, however, rejected as unsuitable but as having, in our opinion, a less pressing claim in open competition; some are rejected because they do not seem particularly outstanding and have already received a good offer from elsewhere.

The case to be made for giving weight to non-academic factors is strong indeed, and the system probably fails to accommodate satisfactorily to these factors. The slender case for deciding entry only on grades is illustrated by a Schools Council report which found that:

> The distinction between the lower boundary of grade B and the upper boundary of grade D, although crucial for many candidates aspiring to enter higher education, can hardly be described as significant in terms of attainments represented by those boundaries.

But this fact must be considered against the background that the great majority of candidates entering medicine handsomely surpass minimum academic requirements and are at the same time people of wide accomplishment and good potential. The problem is not that many unsuitable people are admitted to read medicine but that many who are well suited cannot be admitted.

There is less point in having interviews if some of the questions are not searching. It is both relevant and appropriate to explore whether individuals have begun to think about possible conflicts between a career in medicine and their own personal lives, their beliefs, and their wider interests. Medical schools are criticised for not helping applicants to acquire insight into the realities of the education, training, and career, and at the same time are criticised

Interviews and offers

if they use an interview to confront applicants with some of the possible tensions ahead—tensions which for some are a potent cause of later disillusionment with their career. The problem is that any such question is so often interpreted by unsuccessful applicants as discrimination and the reason for rejection. Not so: the answers are neither right nor wrong, just an indication of the development of an honest, thoughtful point of view.

Interviewers are chosen both from teachers of the sciences basic to medicine (who may or may not be medically qualified themselves) and from practising doctors who teach clinical medicine, as whole time academics, as consultants, or as general practitioners who are part time teachers. Some schools assemble a large group to interview each candidate; we prefer a small, more informal group.

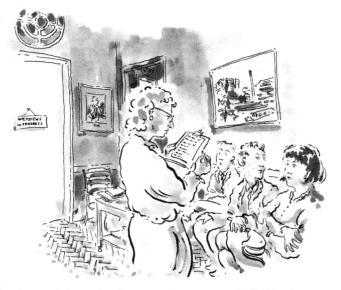

Members of interviewing panels serve as individuals, not as representatives of particular specialties. They know that medicine offers wide career opportunities; that most doctors will end up looking after patients but that not all do; that more will work outside hospitals than inside; that both the training and the job itself are demanding physically and emotionally. They also know that whatever the final occupation of a doctor his training entails the need to make decisions (often on incomplete evidence) and to communicate with patients while at the same time attaining and maintaining moderately exacting academic standards. The aim is not to pick men and women for specific tasks but to train wise, bright, humane, multipotential individuals who will find a niche somewhere in medicine.

48

After each interview our panel members individually grade the candidate as A (make an offer), B^1 (make an offer if the competition and number of places left allow, otherwise put on waiting list), B^2 (waiting list, to be reconsidered after the A level results), and C (reject). The panel then agrees its overall decision and the chairman explains and if necessary amplifies each decision to the dean within 24 hours of the interview. On the rare occasions that the panel is unable to agree the decision is left to the admission tutor or dean.

An offer made to an applicant who has already achieved the minimum academic requirement is unconditional. All candidates who have already attained the minimum grades required at first attempt cannot automatically receive a place because far more applicants reach this standard than the school can take. We make offers on all round merit and potential as best we can assess them on all the evidence. If the A level examinations have yet to be taken an offer is conditional on the applicant obtaining these grades at the first attempt. We occasionally set a higher target to an applicant who seems in need of an incentive to work, but he or she would normally be accepted with the minimum. Sometimes a lower than normal minimum target is set either to take the pressure off candidates working under unfavourable circumstances or to attract an outstanding applicant.

Some medical schools take the highest grades as the final arbiter of admission. Others (see table I, p 21) use grades primarily to ensure sufficient academic ability, although most entrants to these schools achieve substantially higher grades than the minimum requirements. Very few students indeed are accepted to read medicine in the UK with A level grades below an average of CCC. The mean A level score of entrants is ABB. Most schools require higher grades if candidates retake A levels—for example, they may require an A in chemistry and two B grades instead of a B in chemistry and two C grades if a further year of study is undertaken. When examinations are repeated within only a few months the target is likely to be intermediate between the original requirement and that for a year later.

Finally, applicants must remember that achievement of minimum grades at first attempt (or higher grades subsequently) does no more than qualify them to enter the real competition. No level of A level achievement gives entitlement to a place without consideration of other factors. Many more applicants can obtain the necessary grades than can possibly be taken under a fixed quota system. All medical schools try very hard to be fair but a number of able applicants will inevitably be disappointed.

Starting medicine:
the basic medical sciences course

The medical schools accept only the most gifted students and then expose them to an educational process so rigid in its structure and limited in its horizons that at graduation the medical student is the best informed but most poorly educated of all graduates. This system, which is designed to eliminate the incompetent, also often succeeds in stifling the inventiveness and imagination of the most competent and signally fails to develop those intellectual attitudes necessary for continuing self-education.

D C EVERED AND H D WILLIAMS (1980)

The making of a physician is primarily an educational and not a professional question ... he must be trained not only in the observation of facts but also in the habit of handling them—in a word, in methods of reasoning which alone supply any solution to the problems of professional life.

CHARLES WILSON (later Lord Moran) (1932)

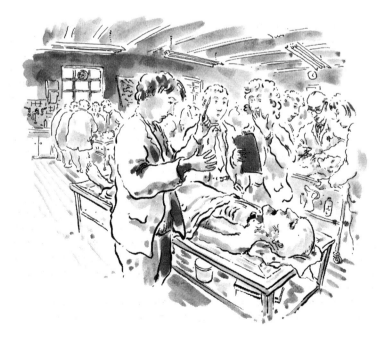

The basic medical sciences course

The first few weeks at medical school are bewildering. The first two years are filled with facts, sometimes heavy going, and in many schools a little tantalising for those who are understandably impatient to get to grips with patients and disease. Although there is much to learn there is no excuse for it being dull. Courses are currently in a ferment of reform. In a few years all will be focused on the ability to relate, think, question, and solve rather than to absorb facts like a sponge. The biological and behavioural sciences basic to medicine will be taught in relation to the need to know and understand about health care in general and clinical medicine in particular. Consequently the traditional divide between "preclinical" and "clinical" will increasingly become blurred until it disappears altogether.

Anatomy, the structure of the human body (including embryology, its process of development); physiology, the normal function; biochemistry, the chemistry of body processes; pharmacology, the properties and metabolism of drugs in the body; psychology and sociology, the basis of human behaviour; and general pathology, the general principles of the mechanisms of disease, form the core of the first two years' work. The extent to which this instruction is integrated with and taught through glimpses of patients and their disease differs between schools.

THE SUBJECTS TAUGHT

Anatomy is taught partly by dissection of dead bodies (cadavers), partly by the use of microscope slides, and partly as a living subject using models or patients. It is no longer necessary for students to own a microscope. At many schools students dissect the whole body in groups over one year, working on one part at a time: arm, chest, head and neck, leg, and abdomen. The dissecting room is an unpleasant shock at first but not for long.

Tutorials and closed circuit television demonstrations in the dissecting room are used to guide dissection, and progress is checked and consolidated by frequent oral examinations. Surface anatomy in living people and radiological anatomy are components of all courses. Dissection may seem to waste time when only one or two in each group of students can be dissecting at once, but it is a well tried method of learning; some schools now teach all except the most important areas by demonstration of prosected specimens and not by dissection. Preserved cadavers make for difficult dissection; fortunately much of the knowledge of anatomy necessary for clinical practice is revised and extended later by assisting at surgical operations.

Other subjects are taught by lectures, laboratory practicals, demonstrations, films, tutorials, and projects. Often students per-

The basic medical sciences course

form simple tests on themselves under supervision in physiology and pharmacology practicals; it is a good way both to learn and to begin to appreciate what patients endure. Projects help to develop the ability to think, to reason, and to escape from the forced feeding of fact which forms too large a part of traditional medical courses and tends to stifle curiosity. Project work also makes it necessary to discover how to make full use of the library. The only substantial opportunity for supervised laboratory research in the preclinical years comes from honours courses that are either an integral part of the course or intercalated (see below).

Preclinical courses are gradually becoming more coordinated and more specifically directed towards the vocational aspects of medicine. Each subject has a central core of knowledge special to itself but once that has been outlined there is much to be said for teaching structure and function simultaneously, building up knowledge body system by body system. For example, it is logical to teach together the anatomy and physiology of the heart and circulatory system. Normal function is often best understood by its breakdown in disease, as for example in inherited metabolic diseases, and here the clinician can make a valuable contribution to preclinical teaching by discussing and demonstrating patients as examples.

TUTORS, TEACHERS, AND ASSESSMENTS

Tutorial teaching in small groups supplements larger group teaching and gives a better opportunity to question and discuss. Many schools also have a coordinating tutor or vice dean to students on the preclinical course who keeps an eye on their overall academic programme and progress during the first two or three years of the course. Students may also have a personal tutor, a member of staff detailed to be a friend and adviser. The success or failure of the personal tutor system depends on the individuals concerned. On the whole students seem to prefer to obtain personal advice from sympathetic staff members with whom they have day by day contact during the course rather than to seek out a contrived adviser with whom there may be no natural contact. In many schools students also play a part in befriending other students—for example, a second year student may take some responsibility for a first year student, and a clinical student for a preclinical student.

The form of the preclinical course probably matters much less than the quality and enthusiasm of its teachers. No particular curriculum has been proved better than others, not least because it is far from clear when and how to measure success. Creating and sustaining interest and stimulating critical thought are in my view the most important goals. Interest is best sustained by showing the clinical relevance of science to medicine; a preclinical student commented that "examples of clinical applications give you enough energy and curiosity to keep going for another couple of weeks."

The balance between continuous assessment during the course and major examinations at the end of the year varies considerably. Students at traditional schools which rely almost completely on an end of year examination usually wish that more credit were given to performance during the course. Students at schools which have largely replaced major examinations by continuous assessment complain instead about the stress and strain of frequent tests throughout the year. It is a matter of individual preference.

Around 7% of medical students fail to complete the course. Most fail at the end of the first year (because of misjudgment of the amount of work necessary, failure to learn to organise their own work, a waning of motivation, or because of the diversion of personal entanglements). A few fail at the end of the second year. If examinations held in June of each of the first two years are failed they must be passed at second attempt in September. Students rarely drop out in the clinical years: a change of heart or illness are the usual reasons.

INTERCALATED HONOURS DEGREES

An increasing number of students at schools with a two year preclinical course now undertake an intercalated BSc honours degree in a third preclinical year. Their contemporaries go straight into the clinical course. A wide range of BSc courses is available in different schools and includes single subject courses in a preclinical science department or a combination of course units in different departments, such as "infection and immunity" courses mounted jointly by departments of medical microbiology and immunology. London University students can arrange to undertake an intercalated BSc in a college other than their own medical school.

There are several attractions of taking an intercalated BSc degree which more than outweigh the disadvantage of losing immediate contact with colleagues with whom the first two years have been spent and on lengthening the course by one year. The advantages include the development of a critical approach, a training in laboratory and library research procedures, and education in depth in a field of science often chosen to have direct relevance to the understanding of clinical medicine. It is useful to have a BSc degree to mark the years of study of sciences related to medicine because it provides a qualification which most students do not have when they enter the keen competition for postgraduate training posts. A science degree is also useful to the occasional student who drops out of the medical course and would otherwise have nothing to show for several years of university work. Clinical teachers used to regard an intercalated BSc as irrelevant to clinical training, but this attitude is passing, not least because of the increasing relevance of the subjects of BSc courses to the understanding of disease.

A new BSc course in clinical science, which is normally taken between the second and third clinical years, started in London University in 1987, based for all medical students of the university at St Mary's Hospital Medical School and mounted jointly by St Mary's Hospital Medical School, the Royal Postgraduate Medical School, and Imperial College. The course covers information science, logic, molecular biology, membrane physiology, and bioengineering and is particularly designed to give an appropriate background to those interested in clinical research. Several medical schools are now following this lead, either under the title BSc in clinical science or as a BMedSci, which is how Newcastle University had long described its intercalated bachelor's degrees during the medical course, regardless of whether they have focused primarily on basic medical science or on clinical science. Nottingham University routinely awards a BMedSci to all successful medical students after three years (see p 29).

The major problem about intercalated BSc courses is that they are only covered by mandatory local authority grants for students whose homes are in Scotland and Northern Ireland. It seems to fly in the face of equal opportunities that those whose homes are in England and Wales have to pay the fees and support themselves for that year unless they are fortunate enough to obtain a discretionary grant. Several scholarships are available at all schools and fees are set at the relatively low "self funded student" level but many students are faced with a difficult financial situation. On the whole it is a sacrifice worth making—for parents as well as students, but clearly the situation is unsatisfactory, and eligibility for a mandatory grant should be extended to all home students.

It is difficult to get the feel of what it is like to be a preclinical student from dry description of the course itself, so the chapter ends with two student glimpses, one of a day in her life on a traditional course, and the other of the introduction to training in listening to and talking with patients at the time of transition between the preclinical and clinical courses.

A day in the life of a preclinical student

Our working day begins at 9 am with a lecture. Today we start with physiology and a lecture on respiratory function, peppered with complex graphs and slides full of figures. All through the hour, which seems a long one, my stomach rumbles loudly. I have had to go without breakfast

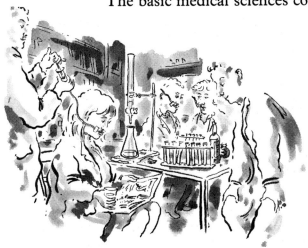

because today's physiology practical demands a 12 hour fast. I must avoid the restaurant, as the temptation to have coffee and a bun would be overpowering.

After the lecture I slip on a lab coat and go to the physiology laboratory to reread the instructions for the practical. Four volunteers are required to swallow nasogastric tubes. I try to decide whether I will volunteer. When the whole class is assembled it transpires that only four of us have fasted, so there is little choice. The demonstrator sprays my right nostril with local anaesthetic and pours me a glass of iced water. As I swallow the water through a straw he pushes the tube (which is quite narrow) into my nose and down my throat. It is not nearly so bad as I had expected and I manage without undue embarrassment. The tube is inserted up to a mark and the end taped to my cheek. I am then given a tablet to swallow. It is an antihistamine agent to prevent side effects from the injection of histamine which I will be given in 15 minutes. Of the other three "volunteers" one is given an injection of a hormone called gastrin, one a hot Bovril drink, and one a large glass of sherry (on an empty stomach too).

The experiment necessitates measuring the output of gastric acid after the administration of these stimulants to see which elicits the greatest response. It is important that no extra substance is swallowed, so that I have to spit out all my saliva into a beaker, which I carry sorrowfully around the lab with me. No chance of keeping one's dignity in this practical. The other members of my group titrate the acid removed from my stomach and work out all the figures.

At last, after almost three hours, all the readings have been taken and I can remove the tube. This is far worse than swallowing it but it is a relief to get rid of the irritation in my throat caused by the tube.

After the class, I rush down to the restaurant and eat a huge lunch. The experiment has not spoilt my appetite. After lunch there is the weekly anatomy viva, so I spend some time (as do many others) in the library going over details. Anatomy vivas dominate our thoughts from week to week. We do most of the weekly dissection in one day; six days later we are formally examined on all the minutiae we were supposed to have found at dissection.

The basic medical sciences course

Each group sits round its cadaver, trembling, and a member of staff sits at the head (literally) and goes round each one in turn for an agonising 30 minutes. It can be a most uncomfortable experience if you have not done enough work. This week the ordeal centres on the muscles, nerves, and blood supply of the forearm. Today we get off to a bad start when our group's wiseguy cracks a joke which is not appreciated by the lecturer. So we are asked everything in the finest detail and are found wanting.

After the viva refreshment is the main need, and we repair to the restaurant for tea and the inevitable "post mortem" on our performance. At 4 pm I attend a lecture on the anatomy of the hand, which I shall dissect tomorrow. The lecturer goes very fast and I give up trying to take notes.

Normally I go straight home to eat, but this evening I am going to an entertainment laid on by the drama and literary societies, so I work for an hour and then eat in the hospital. The concert is great fun, combining drama, poetry readings (not the stodgy kind), and songs. I get home just after 11 pm and fall into bed.

KATE WISHART

Communication skills

You will be spending the rest of your prospective career talking to patients so it's nice to be able to do it well—indeed it's one of the major ways in which your medical skills are judged. To this end, the communication skills teaching is designed to give you a few pointers as to how to handle various patient scenarios so that you and the patient go away happy (and less liable to sue!).

There is a small group of students, a doctor, psychologist, and a TV/video at each session. You are in the room next door with an actor and a video camera to keep you company. Before it starts, all you can think of are your friends watching you on TV next door in this totally artificial situation and how stupid it all seems! But then the actor arrives playing your patient and you're away. They might be trying to tell you about their piles, or of "trouble down below, Doctor." They may be a shy, retiring nun or the Marquis de Sade—anything is fair game. There are various scenarios and patients that the actors can play and they are invariably superb. You forget it's all a sham and that your friends are next door watching you on TV.

A particular favourite that you are asked to do is explain to a patient (actor) a special test he or she needs to have done and what it will be like for him or her. The old chestnut is endoscopy. This usually leads to some wonderful descriptions of TV cameras being forced down the unfortunate patient's throat which, judging by their aghast expressions, seems to conjure up images of the cameraman, floor manager, and producer going down to have a look, too! The most difficult to explain are tests involving the injection of a harmless radioactive isotope. On at least one occasion the patient left the room convinced his hair would fall out and his skin peel and blister in a most Chernobyl-esque manner!

After the consultation you go back next door and receive comments from those watching. Emphasis is put on your good points as well as your goofs, so it boosts your confidence (that's half the trick in good communication) for dealing with real patients, as well as raising your awareness of the possible pitfalls. Invaluable skills are learned which past students—now doctors—say they are still using on the wards now.

LIZ JAMES

The clinical years

Two things make medical students work: one is exams, the other is patients.

WILLIAM SUMMERSKILL (1980)

The piercing and intelligent recognition and appreciation of minor differences is the real essential factor in all successful medical diagnoses. Eyes and ears which can see and hear, memory to record at once and recall at pleasure the impression of the senses, and an imagination capable of weaving a theory or piecing together a broken chain or unravelling a tangled clue.

JOSEPH BELL (nineteenth century) teacher of Arthur Conan Doyle and role model for Sherlock Holmes

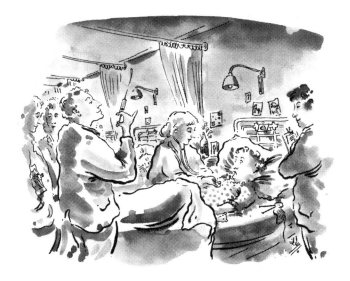

Students suddenly emerge from what may sometimes seem to be two years of non-clinical frustration into an apparently bright and exciting world of clinical medicine, a world which all too easily collapses in a sense of anticlimax. The anticlimax occurs partly because the pace of teaching suddenly slows and method and approach become more important than fact. Learning is from patients with a haphazard selection of diseases and not from well

57

structured courses. Teaching is geared to helping students discover for themselves and is only an intermittent refinement and gloss on the product of the student's own initiative and application. More importantly, the anticlimax may be because getting alongside patients who are ill and often tired may not be easy and some students find it very hard.

Clinical education is a composite of learning facts, acquiring practical skills, taking responsibility, and developing the ability to make decisions. Medicine is a curious mixture of art and science, its clinical bedside method a sharp contrast to the exactness of science and to the complexity of laboratory and radiological investigation. Yet failure to become competent at this stage in listening to and examining patients may result in failure ever to acquire a solid foundation in practical clinical skills. At this early stage of the course there is time to practise unsophisticated but in fact not so simple skills over and over again without great pressure to amass a pile of detailed theoretical knowledge of disease.

Several schools start the clinical course with a nursing attachment, a most appropriate introduction to clinical medicine. For one week each student keeps the hours of a nurse and undertakes the same duties, learning the ward routine and discovering the teamwork essential to good medical care. The nursing week ensures that future generations of doctors will be under no misapprehension about the vital importance of continuous observation, sympathy and encouragement and will not be deluded into thinking that patients in hospital are kept clean, tidy, fed, and cooperative without a great deal of effort. This introduction should help to stifle at birth any temptation to medical arrogance.

Medical students have much to learn from nurses; even as recently qualified doctors they learn to rely heavily on the judgment and experience of the ward sister. The sister in charge of the ward is a key person in every clinical student's life (sometimes *for* life, but that's another matter). Time spent in developing a harmonious working relationship is time well spent.

There is a tendency to react to what may seem to be a slow and pedestrian start to clinical medicine either by indulging, to the detriment of attendance on the wards, in all the sparetime pursuits dropped on the approach to the 2nd MB or by withdrawing into the library. The practical skills of medicine can no more be acquired by reading books than a driving test can be passed by studying the Highway Code. Sometimes students are discouraged by having to wait around for their teachers; neither teachers nor students should keep the other waiting. It is true that teachers have a normal day's clinical work to fit in around their teaching and that emergencies upset the best laid plans, but the remedy is largely one of good organisation.

THE FIRM

Most clinical teaching is arranged by attachment of a group of students to a clinical "firm" for apprentice-type training on the hospital wards. Firms differ considerably in structure according to specialty and hospital but a medical or surgical firm may typically consist of one or two consultant physicians or surgeons, a senior registrar (the preconsultant stage of training) or a registrar (the first stage of specialist training), a senior house officer (who has completed at least two house officer posts after qualification), and one or two preregistration house officers, who are in their first year of supervised practical training immediately after passing the MB degree.

By a strange accident of history physicians—that is, doctors practising medicine not surgery—are in Britain called "Dr" while surgeons (except in Scotland) pride themselves on being called "Mr," although they too have the same university MB qualification which entitles them to the courtesy title of "Dr." The "Mr" convention is a form of inverted snobbery. For centuries physicians had a university education and looked down on surgeons, who as craftsmen were not accepted as members of a learned profession; this happened despite the lonely pleas of more enlightened members of the profession such as John Gregory, professor of medicine at Edinburgh, who wrote in 1771 with respect to surgeons, physicians, and apothecaries:

> As a doctor's degree can never confer sense, the title alone can never command regard; neither should the want of it deprive any man of the esteem and deference due to real merit.

When, in the last century, surgery became accepted as a full part of medicine in its widest sense, and the same basic medical qualifications became necessary for physicians and surgeons, surgeons proudly retained the title of "Mr" and have done so ever since. Scottish surgeons, however, tend to prefer to be called "Dr."

The firm admits patients partly from the outpatient clinics, to which patients are referred by their general practitioners for a second opinion, and partly from among those admitted directly as emergency cases at the request of a general practitioner or through the accident and emergency department from the street. The firms in a specialty divide up the week between them so that one firm is always on duty to receive emergency cases (emergency intake or "on take") night and day, weekday and weekend. When on take all the firm except the consultant but including one of the students lives in the hospital; the consultant is available by telephone when not in the hospital. Intake duty is an excellent opportunity to learn

The clinical years

because students see new patients and are taught hour by hour as acute conditions develop and problems unravel.

Each patient in hospital (inpatient) is allocated to a student. The number of students on each firm should not be so great that each student is responsible for fewer than four patients at any time, which means that the optimum number of students per firm is usually about five. The students learn primarily by "clerking" their own patients—that is, making notes of what the patient has noticed about the illness (the clinical history), by examining the patient fully (to discover the physical signs), and by following the patient's progress day by day, noting any change in the symptoms and signs, the results of investigations, and the treatment given.

If the patient has special investigations the student attends, if the patient has an operation the student assists in the operating theatre, and if the patient has a baby the student delivers it. Assisting in theatre generally means holding the wound open with retractors and cutting stitches. Students take blood from patients for tests, a chore which they sometimes resent but which enables them to develop a skill while contributing to the patient's care.

Far from considering a student to be an invasion of their privacy most patients appreciate the interest and friendship of their "young doctor," except perhaps when he or she is very new and armed with a syringe and needle. Patients are pleased to have someone at hand who has more time than the doctors and nurses to explain, sympathise, and encourage, and they are diverted by taking an interest in the hopes and prospects of "their" student. Both students and their critics outside hospital often fail to give due credit for the valuable contribution which medical students make to patients' welfare, a contribution which requires time, trouble, and sensitivity. Students may also directly help in the assessment and management of their patients by discovering details about the history of the illness or by being the first to notice new developments. The questions and comments of students also keep the doctors on their toes.

TEACHING

Teaching on the firm takes place partly on ward rounds, partly in seminars, and partly in the outpatient clinics. Each consultant probably does two "business" rounds each week, on which the patients under his care are re-examined and discussed with the registrar and house officers. Another round is likely to be devoted entirely to teaching and testing the students on the patients under their care. The registrar or senior registrar teaches formally at least once a week besides minute by minute teaching of the student on emergency intake and is available to answer questions informally day by day about any of a student's allocated patients.

Larger group teaching takes place in clinical meetings (sometimes known by their North American name of grand rounds), radiology meetings (at which the week's x ray films are discussed with the radiologist), and histopathology meetings, when the structure of tissue removed at biopsy or operation is shown by the pathologist and discussed. When patients die a postmortem examination is carried out by a pathologist, if the relatives agree, and both students and doctors are able to confirm and extend the diagnosis made in life.

All in all there is much going on but students need to participate actively if they are to learn as much as they can. Each condition needs to be read up when it is seen and a note kept of the diseases covered so that gaps can be filled in by reading later. During clinical training it simply is not feasible to see patients with all the conditions about which some knowledge is expected, and no reasonable examiner expects a student either to have seen or to know everything.

Reading is made much more interesting if textbooks are supplemented by a regular look at editorial articles in the three major weekly general medical journals, the *British Medical Journal*, *The Lancet*, and the *New England Journal of Medicine*. The editorials are readable, concise discussions of new or controversial aspects of important conditions. Examiners read the same editorials (some write them and would be flattered to be both read and remembered).

THE SPECIALTIES TAUGHT

Students normally spend two or three months each on a surgical and a medical firm at the beginning of the clinical course and a similar period towards the end. Clinical medicine is learnt best through taking responsibility. One of the most valuable experiences is to undertake towards the end of clinical training one or more "shadow" house officer posts in medicine, surgery, or obstetrics, each for two or four weeks; this is best done on a firm which has no other students at the time, which usually means going to a hospital distant from the main teaching hospital. The shadow understudies the house officer, taking personal responsibility for the day to day care of a few patients (under supervision), and quickly learns practical procedures such as setting up intravenous infusions and bladder catheterisation. A similar but more taxing assignment is to stand in for a house officer as a student assistant at a time of holiday or sickness; students are paid for undertaking these assistantships.

The clinical years

About three months of the clinical course are occupied with pathology, which includes clinical biochemistry (the biochemistry of disease), histopathology (the microscopic structure of diseased tissues), haematology (the study of diseases affecting blood and bone marrow), microbiology (including the study of bacteria and viruses), and immunology (the role of immunity in disease). Without a knowledge of disease processes it is very difficult to understand and to interpret clinical signs and symptoms. The blood, body fluids, and tissue samples taken from patients in the course of diagnosing their illnesses are analysed in pathology laboratories. Pathology in relation to sudden death or death in suspicious circumstances is the basis of forensic medicine, which also embraces the relationship between medicine and the law, an aspect of medical training usually included in the pathology teaching.

The other major clinical specialties—obstetrics (the care of pregnant women) and gynaecology (the specialty devoted to diseases confined to women); paediatrics (child health); and psychiatry (the care of patients with mental illness)—are also taught by attachment to firms.

Other specialties occupy a smaller part of the students' time and are taught primarily by attendance at outpatient clinics, teaching rounds, lectures, and demonstrations. General understanding of these "minor" specialties is expected rather than much detailed knowledge: they include neurology (disorders of motor and sensory function of the brain, spinal cord, and peripheral nerves); rheumatology and rehabilitation, alias physical medicine (medical disorders of joints, such as arthritis, and rehabilitation of patients with physical disabilities); genitourinary medicine, alias venereology (sexually transmitted diseases); dermatology (skin diseases); geriatrics (the care of the elderly); ophthalmology (eye diseases); otolaryngology, more easily remembered as ENT (disorders of ear, nose, and throat); orthopaedics (disorders of bones and joints requiring surgery); urology (conditions of the kidneys, ureters, and bladder amenable to surgical treatment); and anaesthetics. These many specialties can easily turn the curriculum into a disjointed hotchpotch and so far as possible their teaching is integrated into the major medical and surgical teaching firms.

Attachments to an accident and emergency department are popular because they entail contact with a wide variety of conditions. Students see new patients in the front line and feel at last that they are doing something useful by stitching wounds and undertaking other minor procedures.

An increasing amount of teaching takes place out of hospital, notably in general practice and community medicine. Newer schools such as Southampton, Nottingham, and Leicester tend to put a larger emphasis on teaching outside hospital than many older schools. The purpose is not to train medical students to become general practitioners (although half of the students will eventually go into general practice) but to show in surgeries and in patients' own homes a different spectrum of disease, an approach appropriate to handling patients with minor everyday illnesses, and the different pattern of working conditions outside hospital. Insight, not instruction, is the keynote, a counterbalance to the rarified atmosphere of hospital, an awareness essential for all those concerned with partnership of care between hospital and general practice. Public health medicine and community health are specialties concerned with the prevention of disease and with the health of populations; planning of health services outside hospital is one important aspect of its work.

ELECTIVES

The curriculum might well seem overcrowded with too little opportunity for individual preference, interest, and experience. This generally is so. One university, Southampton, attempts to overcome this criticism by devoting the major part of the fourth year (the second clinical year) to a project. Most schools offer a shorter elective period (usually two or three months) in which students may undertake any medically related study at home or abroad. Most students take the opportunity to see medicine in a different setting in another country and often obtain practical experience at the same time. Some take the opportunity to repeat parts of the curriculum or to obtain further experience of particular specialties which interest them but play only a minor part in the undergraduate course, such as radiology or mental handicap. The *British Medical Journal* offers a different sort of opportunity through competitive elective studentships designed to provide insights into medical journalism.

ASSESSMENTS

Schools adopt different systems of assessing students' clinical progress. Most still put the major emphasis on a final MB examination divided into two sections: pathology, taken 6–12 months before the end of the clinical course, and medicine, surgery, obstetrics and gynaecology, and clinical pharmacology and therapeutics, taken together at the end. The important conditions covered in the "minor" specialty attachments are included in the major subjects. An increasing number of medical schools now have the written examination for Finals a year before the clinicals, to encourage concentration on clinical skills before becoming house officers.

The clinical years

The final MB examination comprises multiple choice questions, essay questions, and practical examinations. The examinations in medicine, surgery, and obstetrics and gynaecology put most emphasis on clinical examinations at the bedside, which test practical skills in talking to patients, examining them, and making a diagnosis. Oral examinations are also held. However brilliant their theoretical knowledge, students generally cannot pass the final MB if they fail a clinical examination.

Students are also assessed on their performance in each part of the course, sometimes by a practical or written examination. These assessments are used to certify satisfactory completion of the course and do not contribute to the mark in the final MB at most schools. Nevertheless, all parts of the course must be satisfactorily completed before students are allowed to enter the final MB examination. Some schools, such as Birmingham, give greater weight than other schools to continuous assessment in relation to finals.

Although it may be difficult to get the feel of what it is like to be a preclinical student without an account of a typical day, it is doubly difficult to shadow the clinical student, whose activities are both different from those of other students and diverse. So some St Mary's students have contributed the following accounts. The first describes a day on a surgical firm, an experience not so different from that of the house officer, except of course in respect to the responsibility carried. The second is a day in general practice, the third concerns a night in the accident and emergency unit, and the fourth a first night on obstetrics. Finally, a more exotic day on elective.

A day in the life of a clinical student in hospital

A rude awakening by alarm clock. Will I ever get used to 8 am ward rounds? I arrive a few minutes before the surgical registrar and just have time to say a quick good morning to "my" patients. (Patients are allocated as they come in, by our elected firm leader.) Today is Tuesday, which means that the registrar's round will be followed at 9 am by the consultant's teaching round.

The registrar's round consists of a brisk visit to each patient to check on temperatures, wounds, and drains besides general inquiries about comfort, specific complaints, and a check on the drugs being prescribed.

The little troupe of white coats hurries through the male and female wards and briefly visits a third, which is lodging one of our patients because our own wards are full. Then we go down to the children's ward to see a rather sorrowful little girl who had her appendix out yesterday. The white coats stay a little longer with her—children always get special attention. But I must dash up to the switchboard to collect a bleep and the key of the duty student's room, as it is my turn on take.

The clinical years

9 am and the regiment is complete: the consultant surgeon, exquisitely suited, slick, and awe inspiring; the registrar, hoping he has not forgotten any detail; the senior house officer, keeping a low profile; the houseman, notebook in hand, ready to write down any tests or treatment requested; and six students, desperately rehearsing mentally the details of their own particular patients.

Not all firms are quite like this one, but, then, not all consultants are quite like ours. No one is safe from his penetrating questions. He is a master of discovering the one thing that you don't know, and if he asks you something you *can* answer then he keeps on firing questions at you until you flounder. All in a good cause, though: it is an effective way of fixing facts firmly in the memory.

I survive without mishap today, having only to present a patient with a straightforward hernia. Another is less fortunate. It soon becomes obvious that he has not checked up on his patient before the rounds and he tries to convey the impression that this is an isolated lapse. The consultant, merciless, asks the patient when she last saw the student. Oh dear—not for four days. The poor boy doesn't stand a chance.

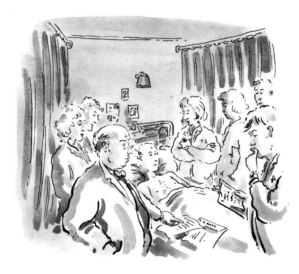

After this ordeal two students go off with the consultant and the registrar to the outpatient clinic. It is my day for taking blood samples from the patients on the wards. Blood taking can be a nightmare at the beginning but the more you do the easier it becomes. It is amazing how many patients have disappearing veins—now you see one, now you don't. We were lucky because our houseman patiently showed us at the beginning how to take blood from tricky veins.

Next on the timetable is the weekly medical meeting at which one or two cases are presented and discussed in the presence of most of the medical

The clinical years

staff and students. One of the cases today is fascinating but the second is way over my head. Lunch follows, but no sooner have I sat down than I hear a bleep which sounds louder than most. Then I realise that the sounds are coming from my own pocket. It takes time to get used to carrying a bleep and I still find that its summons sets the adrenaline going. This time it is the houseman calling to ask me to see a boy in casualty—I can eat my lunch first but he will expect me in five minutes.

The patient, a teenage boy, is too unwell for two people to question and examine him (normally every patient is fully assessed by both student and houseman). He has been knocked down by a car and is admitted for close observation, suspected of having a ruptured spleen.

From casualty I go to the outpatient department to sit in on a urology clinic. Although attached to a general surgical firm we are expected at the same time to learn something of the specialties of urology and orthopaedics. Outpatient clinics are always interesting. One learns a lot about common complaints, and it is enlightening to see how experienced doctors handle their patients.

Immediately after the clinic, I go back to the ward to see the injured lad. The houseman is already there, checking his pulse, blood pressure, and temperature. The boy looks worse and the houseman has asked the registrar to see him again. The registrar remains cautious and advises that blood should be cross matched urgently in case it should be necessary to operate at short notice.

During the evening we are asked to see two more patients in casualty. One seems to be a medical case and is admitted under the physicians; we admit the other to our surgical ward. I also find time to see my own patients again and to stop for a chat with each.

After supper the condition of the injured boy is still deteriorating, and at 10 pm the registrar decides to operate. I "scrub up" and assist by holding retractors and cutting stitches. You get a better view when scrubbed up and learn more by helping. The boy's spleen is indeed ruptured. It is removed and the operation is a success.

At midnight, after a nightcap in the doctors' mess, I am more than ready to go to bed in my room with "Surgical student on take" on the door. My bleep is on the pillow by my ear and I intend to get off to sleep quickly, before it goes off: the houseman has promised faithfully to call me if anything interesting happens. . . .

KATE WISHART

A day in general practice

My practice starts the day with a team meeting. A coffee fix gives everyone time to label the important events of the next few days. The builders are in, so all hearts will have a continuous murmur today; a new software package will be demonstrated to allow current problems to be highlighted whilst listing previous diagnoses, but will it really help? Instantly I am involved, my opinion sought in a warm welcome to the group. I ask what book I should read to learn about general practice and am told *Middlemarch* by George Eliot. Six months later, having read the book, I am still thinking about what was meant by that answer. In return, they ask me what skills a doctor should have in general practice. Everyone joins in, and the discussion leads us into seeing the patients.

Today I see the patients on my own first. I receive more trust and responsibility from these doctors in a week than in a year at the hospital. Presenting the complaint and my thoughts to the GP is excellent practice at developing a "problem-oriented approach". I am daunted by the impossibility of knowing the person and their history in 10 minutes, and hospital clerkings are little preparation. The long relationship between GP and patient is such a privilege and opportunity for appropriate intervention relevant to the patient's needs and wishes.

I think through the messages I learned from watching myself on video being "consulted" by actors, back at the St Mary's department of general practice. The skills are those of good listening, while considering the possible background to the presenting problem—the family problems, alcoholism—and the needs, articulated or unspoken, for caring, a further specialist opinion, or a prescription. I remember the advice that a holistic viewpoint, and the availability of complementary therapies, can obviate the need for drugs as psychological props for either doctor or patient.

Mr A has low back pain and was given short shrift by the orthopaedic consultant for not having sciatica that would be worth operating on, entirely ignoring his pain. We talk about his weight, posture, and stress at work and re-emphasise his need for exercises and a good chair, which seems more appropriate. Ms B comes in with severe abdominal pain and iliac fossa pain and rebound tenderness. My excitement at a possible hospital referral dies down as the doctor reassures both of us that this is constipation. The case mix is so different in a teaching hospital; a sense of proportion is vital and can only come with experience. Mr C was found to be hypertensive opportunistically at a previous visit, and the nurse has confirmed this subsequently. We discuss what this implies for his future health and treatment, and the doctor and I talk afterwards about current concepts in the management of blood pressure from both personal care and population health perspectives. Every person is different, and requires integrating an understanding of the possible pathologies with what is realistic in their life. Without time or fast investigations nearly every diagnosis may be provisional; "come back tomorrow" is not a cop-out but good management.

In the corridor we have a "kerbside" case conference about what to do with Ms X. She has many problems, and all the partners have been to visit her at one time or other. The latest news is not good, and, although she has heart failure, it is her mobility and risk of hip fracture that we worry about. We visit her before lunch, assess her cardiovascular and neurological status, and find out how well the carers are coping. It may be that improving the lighting will counter her drowsiness and prevent a disastrous fall.

Over lunch we discuss strategies and priorities in looking after someone with diabetes, and the implications for general practitioners of the new NHS changes. The balance has swung away from clinical freedom; doctors have lost much control over their time and decisions, but to quite an extent are being forced to do what they would have liked to do anyway, namely more work on prevention and health promotion. Computerisation has been unavoidable, but as yet wastes far more time than it saves. There

The clinical years

is great potential for clear presentation of patient information and for networking outcomes between patients and practices for audit and research. I sit in quietly as another partner runs a yoga class in her lunchbreak, and feel greatly refreshed for the afternoon.

Later on, I join the local community psychiatric nurse. One of the people we visit has panic attacks when she goes outside. The nurse has given her mental exercises to do at home, and a routine to use when she feels the panic attack developing. We take her out for a walk calmly, and get along without her anxiety becoming panic, which encourages her greatly. Another woman has gradually become more depressed since her husband died, and the nurse is delighted that she has a chance to intervene with counselling and cognitive therapy before a doctor (not from my practice!) has filled her full of tricyclic antidepressants. A third has Alzheimer's disease, and the issue is whether she will leave the frying pan on and burn the house down while her son is out at work.

Back at the practice I get on my bike to go home, overwhelmed by the breadth of insight needed in this work. The loneliness in the consulting room is more than compensated by the warmth of genuine teamwork and equal exchange of views and approaches. Humanity and pathophysiology do mix after all.

TOM ALLPORT

A night in casualty

The night starts with routine handover when the outgoing day staff update the incoming staff on what's been happening all day, which patients are still in the department, and of course how long the waiting time is! Then the influx begins — a wheezy 60 year old having an asthmatic attack, a 55 year old male with congestive heart failure, a 30 year old diabetic suffering hypoglycaemia – the list goes on, but soon begins to repeat itself. This is the part that in itself could become dull and boring. Of course, you are on the sharp end of medicine, you see people recover as a direct result of your intervention, and you get the satisfaction of seeing them leave healthy and full of gratitude. All this for essentially just doing your job – but then the real fun begins as all too soon the pubs are closing.

This is the busiest time because, among Paddington's cosmopolitan population, spirits are at their height (roughly in proportion to their consumption!). Now your skills as a seamstress are really put to the test or else quickly acquired, as the students are involved as much as possible. Once you've stitched a couple of unfortunate victims back together and are seen to be competent then you're on your own. You'll soon be stitching in your sleep (good preparation for those Junior Doctors' hours!) and waiting for your next challenge.

(Un)fortunately, it's not long in arriving, as the "Red Phone" rings. This is direct from the London Ambulance Service to give advance warning of the impending arrival of a casualty by ambulance. Well, I say advance — you may have as much as 2 minutes to prepare yourself for their arrival! All is very slick and professional though; the designated staff covering the "Crash Room" drop whatever they are doing, don gloves and aprons, and check all equipment is present and working. All of a sudden you find yourself doing the same, as the Consultant drags you in and informs you that he would like you to do the chest compressions! This is when you see teamwork at its best. Even though you are in a potentially terrifying situation, calmness is all around as everybody else knows exactly what to do. Sometimes it works and you see somebody literally come back to life in front of you, sometimes it doesn't – but whatever the outcome, you know that everything possible was done. What is more, you had a hand in it and that is the key to a good learning experience. To feel involved and be useful at such a key moment is surely one of the most positive ways in which to decide that yes, this *is* for me! This degree of involvement and experience is hard to beat so all too soon it's become light again, the shift is over, and it's time to rejoin the dreary old outside world.

JAMES WOOLLEY

First delivery

I was woken up by the sound of my bleep. It was barely 4 am and I had been asleep for less than two hours. By the time I had wearily put on my shoes and rushed to her cubicle, she has already begun to push. Jane, the midwife, decided that there was not time for me to put on a gown, so I just put on the gloves. The mother-to-be began to scream as the contractions became stronger and with each push the baby descended further. I placed my left hand on the head as the crown appeared, to stop it rushing out too quickly, while supporting the mother with my right. I could almost feel my heart thumping against my chest. Any remaining signs of tiredness had now completely disappeared in all the excitement. Here I was minutes away from helping to bring a new life into the world.

It all went so quickly after that. First the baby's head appeared and I pulled it down gently to release the anterior shoulder. The rest appeared to come out all by itself. It was 4.36 am precisely and a big baby boy was born. The mother cried with joy as I placed him on her tummy. It's an amazing feeling. The family wouldn't let me go until they had taken a photograph of me holding him in my arms. By the time I had helped the midwife clear the mess and made sure all was well, it was way past 5 am. Time to get some sleep.

FARHAD ISLAM

A day on elective

Breakfast is pawpaw and aromatic coffee with sacred ibis calling as they fly along the Indian ocean shore. The day starts with the ward round. Eighty kids are packed two or three to a bed. They variously smile or cry, run around fighting or lie listlessly, bellies bulging with kwashiorkor or skin, eyes, and hope flaccid with dehydration. I stride into the measles side ward, a tiny room with three cots now packed with ten mothers and babies in various stages of spottiness.

Admitting a child with measles is easy. The repertoire of a 1 year old is limited to vomiting, diarrhoea, fever, cough, and breathlessness, and with measles all are present in abundance. Red eyes, throat, and eardrums complete the picture examined carefully on the mother's knee (not my own after it was drenched on day one), and the vague but, with experience, characteristic graininess that will pass for a rash on black skin the next day

The clinical years

is hardly needed. The mothers know it to be measles anyway. This is not my benign childhood discomfort of measles. Many of them will die of bronchopneumonia (ampicillin is probably just to keep the doctors happy, but we watch carefully for signs of staphylococci) or of dehydration, which has become my personal crusade. My five minute lecture in broken Swahili attempts to persuade the mother to take on the responsibility of forcing in rehydration fluid tirelessly. So my round of the measles ward is basically to take the temperature and respiratory rate and get a general feeling for each child's health. The sick ones get a closer look that always comes down to not enough water, and so, to the general amusement of all, I'm back on my hobby horse for a bit more negotiating about why the child won't drink, or is not getting enough.

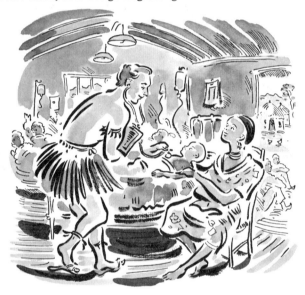

Talking about fluids and measles has been fascinating. Discussions in small groups, wandering round the rickety shacks both in town and out in the surrounding forest, stumble on in Swahili or are translated from Giriama by the wonderful local fieldworker who introduces me. Drunken men lolling in front of their huts accost us and gesticulate aggressively; a group of young women waiting to fill their buckets with water are shy but add their opinions once the most assured has spoken. Water and blood are symbolically related, and when water is drunk they believe it goes into the lungs (hence people with not enough blood, with anaemia, are breathless) and from there round the body in the veins (everyone knows doctors shortcut this by pouring water into the veins direct). Measles, in turn, is within the essence of all people, and must "come out" at some time, inevitably. Vaccines are accepted with equanimity and wry suspension of disbelief in their action. Most dangerous is when the measles goes "back in"—I would explain it as severe dehydration that stops a child's tears, vomit, and diarrhoea—but we agree anyway that death may be imminent.

The clinical years

The ward round continues, from the successes—the child with nephrotic syndrome receiving steroids, whose smile widens daily as his swelling subsides, and the bored happy ones with broken legs hanging from pulleys—to the failures—a paralysed speechless girl brought in after fitting with meningitis for hours, whose family can no longer manage, her living skeleton malnourished and fading away despite all our efforts.

By the end of the ward round the first five or so of the day's 10 or 20 admissions are gathered. Some, at their last gasp for water or air, are given water or blood respectively. The Kenyan medical students amaze me yet again with their skill at slipping needles into the most fragile of dried out baby scalp veins; I amaze myself with a perfect lumbar puncture on a screaming urchin, and take the happily crystal-clear drops off to the laboratory. There I check the results from the day's malaria slides and write the prescriptions accordingly. After a lunch break, I wander into one of the town's cafes, the loose ends on the ward are tied up, and it is time for projects. Rob's is with the high tech transcranial doppler ultrasound measuring blood flow in the middle cerebral artery—will this tell us important things about disease processes in very sick children? The whoosh-whoosh-whoosh pulses out at us as we walk past the little research ward.

My project is to count every drop of fluid going into and out of a child with cerebral malaria over 24 hours. Endlessly there are extra sources of error, not noticed by me as I try to add up volumes and nappy weights in the middle of the night. This year, for better and worse, the rains haven't come properly, so there is little severe malaria, and instead today I can amble back to the guesthouse, luxurious by local standards, for a swim in the balmy buoyant water. There I can dream of my next trip up the coast to the ancient Islamic island city of Lamu, an African Venice of narrow streets, donkeys, cool wind, relaxed gossip, and self indulgence by the waterside.

TOM ALLPORT

Doubts

To write off the whole of medicine as a career would be a serious mistake ... Medicine, especially in the early hospital years, can be very destructive of personal relationships, but the same can be said of the consolidation phase of any occupation. Doctors tend to emphasise the differences from other occupations and ignore the similarities.

MICHAEL PEEL (1993)

One of those crises in which all studies, all intellectual efforts, everything we mean by the life of the mind, appear dubious and devalued and in which we tend to envy every peasant at the plough and every pair of lovers at evening, or every bird singing in a tree and every cicada chirping in the summer grass, because they seem to us to be living such natural, fulfilled and happy lives. We know nothing of their troubles ...

HERMAN HESSE *The Glass Bead Game*

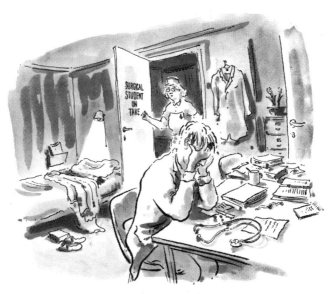

Doubts are a very normal part of life. No university course and no professional training is more likely to raise doubts than medicine: academic doubts, vocational doubts, and personal doubts.

Doubts

Few intending medical students never have reservations about whether medicine is right for them and they for medicine, and those few who have no doubts may perhaps overestimate both their own capability and their suitability. Not many medical students survive five years without wondering if they are on the right road. Few doctors in their first few years escape nagging doubts about the direction in which they would like to go and whether their aspirations are realistic in terms of skills, higher qualifications, and opportunity.

Alongside these various academic and vocational doubts the world of doctors in training also creaks and groans with all the normal difficulties of men and women finding their feet in an adult world. If newly from school they must find accommodation and adjust to life away from home. Mature students must acclimatise to a world that is often very different, more hierarchical, and more juvenile than that in which their feet had already been firmly planted for some years; they also often have to survive greatly reduced financial circumstances. Any one problem or doubt can be coped with, but several simultaneously, together with a course which demands continual concentration and a clear mind, can overwhelm the strongest constitution.

One thing is reasonably certain: decisions either to learn medicine or to abandon the task should not be taken too quickly. As Lilian Hellman wrote in *The Little Foxes*, "Sometimes it's better to let the sun rise again."

ACADEMIC DOUBTS

Academic doubts are probably the easiest of all to resolve. The academic demands of the course and the academic capacity of an individual are susceptible to reasonably objective analysis. The course demands the ability to learn and retain much information and many concepts in different subjects simultaneously and to integrate this learning. An intellect sufficient to achieve at least three C grades in A level science subjects simultaneously at the first attempt with average teaching, together with the ability to persevere, should cope with the medical course without serious difficulty. A determined, well organised person with these academic credentials should not be an academic risk, but more clever people who lack motivation may fail to pass their first or second year examinations.

It is harder for mature students to assess realistically whether or not they have the necessary academic ability for the course, partly because learning does not come so easily after the early 20s and partly because many mature students have little or no background of science. If studying full time they should set themselves a

Doubts

similar standard to those straight from school. If continuing to earn their living while studying part time they may reasonably assemble their A level qualifications piecemeal (so long as each is at a good standard when taken).

One of the saddest sights is the applicant of any age whose academic ability is clearly inadequate for the course but who will not accept that there is no hope. However uncertain the need for a doctor to be clever (and certainly history has shown that a doctor can be successful without being either clever or even safe), the public deserves the best it can get and there are plenty of talented people on offer. Against the competition of more intelligent, equally dedicated, and widely accomplished young men and women, the academically questionable inevitably stand little chance unless possessed of other outstanding qualities. A realistic personal assessment of academic ability is a first necessity in deciding whether medicine is the right choice, a matter of judging correctly the subtle balance between optimism and reality.

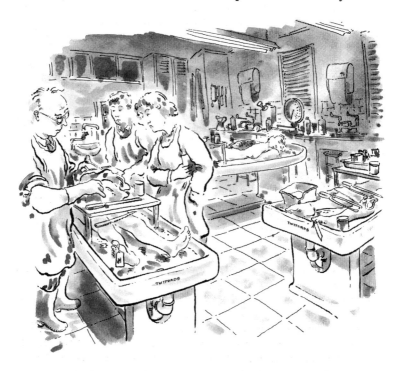

Most academic doubts develop in the preclinical years as a reaction to the apparent irrelevance of much of the course to the goal of clinical medicine. These are not doubts of ability to learn but of patience or commitment. Many of these doubts are the consequence of failure to find out enough at the outset about the course itself. Also it is natural in the first two years to question the ability to endure five years of undergraduate study followed by even more years of postgraduate training.

DEALING WITH PATIENTS

Doubts before and during the preclinical years over whether medicine is the right career are understandable and may partly be avoided by a careful assessment of oneself and the job at the beginning. There may perhaps be no real doubt about academic ability, but what about the ability to handle people sufficiently well and to acquire the necessary practical skills?

There is no way of being absolutely certain of the answers to these questions but indications can be found. Resourceful, practical, sympathetic people who relate easily to others, including those with whom they may disagree, are likely to be suitable. High intelligence is not enough. Those who have taken the trouble to find out what a doctor's work entails by seeing for themselves something of general practice and hospital work and find it attractive have good reason to consider medicine seriously. They might, of course, also be suited to nursing or related careers.

Teachers can help to reinforce motivation by designing undergraduate medical courses which bring together as far as possible science and its clinical applications, keeping the carrot of practical medicine before preclinical students who might otherwise be tempted to abandon their studies, not fully realising how radically preclinical studies differ from clinical medicine.

Learning from patients in the clinical years may be both disturbing and unsettling. Some students have great difficulty in coming to terms with blood, disfigurement, suffering, disability, mental illness, incurable disease, and death. All have some difficulty but most overcome it without becoming hard and completely detached.

A few others find it very difficult to relate to patients. They feel that they are intruding, that they are merely spectators, and they may therefore fail to develop essential skills in talking to and examining patients. Usually the best remedy in these cases is to engineer a greater degree of involvement and responsibility, but teachers need to be perceptive to the need and the student needs determined application. Occasionally this gulf seems unbridgeable, and the student may have to decide whether to change course or to press on to qualification in the knowledge that many careers in medicine are not clinical.

Doubts

TEMPERING STEEL

The importance of seeking help and advice before problems become overwhelming cannot be too strongly emphasised. Most difficulties tend to grow if incubated. In the first place there is no substitute for sharing problems with good friends, and that is one reason why a successful school needs to be a happy, considerate community and not just an academic factory. But the advice of friends may need to be supplemented by tutors, other teachers, doctors in the student health service, pastors, priests, or parents. No problems are unique and none insuperable. Very occasionally the right move is to change course. To change direction for good reason is the beginning of a new opportunity, not a disaster.

Vocational doubts and academic failures occasionally occur during the clinical years because of psychiatric illness, which is sometimes the outcome of relentless parental pressure to follow a career which a student either did not want or for which he or she was unsuited. Depression is the usual response. Expert advice is needed. Psychiatric illness may be self limiting but it may be persistent or recurrent and incompatible with the standards of service and judgment which patients have a right to expect.

The clinical course introduces so many aspects of medicine that it is not surprising that intelligent, self critical students wonder from time to time whether they will ever master enough to qualify let alone to become expert in one discipline while retaining some knowledge of many others. Generations of students have, however, performed very competently as soon as they have been given a job to do as a preregistration houseman, and there is every reason to suppose that future generations will do at least as well.

The overloaded preclinical course is academically stressful, the more so because of the knowledge that failure in end of year examinations and the subsequent resits is final. The clinical course is less taxing academically but far more demanding in human terms. Throughout all these years students are subject to all the other stresses and strains of life, storms which have to be ridden out along with academic and vocational uncertainties. The process is one of tempering steel; most manage very well and emerge able to cope not only with their own problems but with those of their patients.

If comfort is needed, students should from time to time take courage from their good points, which almost invariably outweigh any inadequacy. In the words of Shakespeare in *All's Well that Ends Well*:

> The web of our life is a mingled yarn, good and ill together; our virtues would be proud if our faults whipped them not: and our crimes would despair if they were not cherished by our own virtues.

Qualification and the year
as a preregistration house officer

When I was One
I had just begun

When I was Two
I was nearly new

When I was Three
I was hardly me

When I was Four
I was not much more

When I was Five
I was just alive

But now I am Six, I'm as clever as clever
So I think I'll be Six now for ever and ever.
CHRISTOPHER MEALINGS
(when a final year student,
with apologies to
A A Milne)

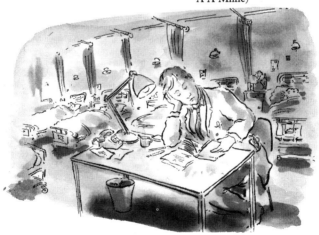

Qualification as a bachelor of medicine and surgery (MB BS or equivalent) after five or six years is not the end but a beginning. Now at last you can learn all the time by doing, a process which continues throughout life; now you are a medical practitioner and can earn your own living. Examinations are not finished and uncertainties about the future are no longer speculations but realities, but at least your first foot is on the ladder. The first rungs are the same for everyone—the preregistration house officer posts,

Qualification

six months in medicine and six months in surgery (or, in a St Mary's scheme, four months each in medicine, surgery, and general practice). These posts must be satisfactorily completed under supervision before a doctor can be fully (rather than provisionally) registered with the General Medical Council and be formally recognised as entitled to embark on postgraduate training. There are preregistration house officer posts in all medium sized and large general hospitals in the United Kingdom.

Whatever else you do or do not do, it is important to complete preregistration posts at the appointed time. It is permissible but unwise, on passing the Final MB, to defer preregistration posts to travel, to undertake more scientific study perhaps leading to a PhD, or even to have a baby. Returning after a break to complete preregistration house officer training is possible but difficult.

THE QUALIFICATIONS

Most students pass the final MB examination (known simply as "finals" or "the MB") at the first attempt; about 10% have to resit all or part of the examination six months later. Very few fail more than once. Candidates who fail the final MB examination or who are ineligible (because they have not undertaken their preclinical studies at a British university) often try to save time at this stage by obtaining a non-university qualification to practise. There have until recently been two of these in England, the LRCS LRCP (Licentiate of the Royal College of Surgeons and Licentiate of the Royal College of Physicians), better known as the "conjoint" because it is organised by the conjoint board of these two royal colleges, and the LMSSA (Licentiate in Medicine and Surgery of the Society of Apothecaries, London), and two in Scotland, set by the Colleges of Physicians and Surgeons in Edinburgh and Glasgow. In future there will be a single non-university licensing examination in medicine, organised jointly by the Royal Colleges in England and Scotland, and by the Society of Apothecaries.

The standard required to pass these examinations is similar to that needed to pass university MB examinations. Most universities will not sponsor their students to take a non-university diploma for longer than the period during which they are permitted to have no more than three consecutive attempts at university finals.

HOUSE JOBS

Medical schools have each built up a pool of preregistration "house jobs," partly posts at the central teaching hospital and other university hospitals in the vicinity and partly posts in hospitals throughout the country, often where graduates of the school are consultants. Applications for these house officer posts are handled centrally by each school; some make a more or less random selection by computer, others match consultants' and students' choices as far as is possible. Not all schools have enough posts for all their graduates, nor do all their graduates seeks posts in the local scheme, as some prefer to find their own posts. There are enough posts for all United Kingdom graduates, and when the number of graduates has increased the number of preregistration house officer posts has been and doubtless will continue to be increased.

Students tend to choose posts at hospitals where they have worked happily as students and to look for consultants who teach conscientiously, take a personal interest in guiding their house officers ("housemen") in their careers, and are pleasant to work for. Sometimes posts are chosen because they are near home or near sailing or some other attraction. On the whole, general experience and responsibility are greater away from the large teaching centres but there is more teaching in the latter.

The amount of supervision, teaching, and experience provided by every preregistration post is assessed formally by the regional postgraduate dean (see p 84) every five years to ensure that it is educationally acceptable. Hours are becoming more standard and shorter, but the pattern of working those hours differs and the work facilities and quality of residential accommodation vary considerably. The most attractive posts generally go to the applicants who not only apply themselves best to their studies but also use their initiative in discovering which are the best jobs.

Men and women are equal as house officers: both are "housemen" and they have identical duties. The only difference in name is between house physicians, who are all "Dr," and house surgeons, who at most hospitals are "Mr," "Mrs," or "Miss." House surgeons sometimes resent losing their hardwon title of "Dr" so soon but their surgical pride soon gains the upper hand.

KINGPIN OF THE FIRM

Housemen are the continuity men and women, the hospital inpatient service's front line contact both with patients and the outside world. This is the final period of their general clinical education and training, but their educational needs too often take second place to long hours on duty and repetitive non-medical tasks, which other members of a well organised team could appropriately do. They are the kingpins of their firms, people who examine all the patients as they arrive day by day, keep the notes, arrange the initial investigations and treatment, prescribe for each

Qualification

minor symptom, keep the intravenous infusions going, and are called by the nursing staff when patients develop new symptoms, signs, or whims, day or night. Housemen also talk to patients' relatives to amplify the history of the illness and to answer the initial anxious questions as well as they can at this early stage of investigation; they may also have the difficult task of being the first to convey bad news. House surgeons assist at their patients' operations and perform a few operations under supervision, such as appendicectomies and stripping varicose veins. They may also have their own operating list for minor operations such as the removal of lumps in the skin.

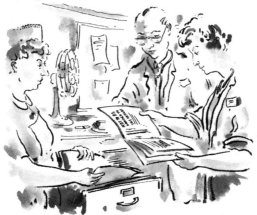

The senior house officer, registrar, or senior registrar checks the houseman's findings, agrees initial treatment, works out a strategy of investigation before the consultant's next visit, or phones him to discuss the situation when matters cannot or should not wait.

Housemen work long hours, but shorter than they did; several measures are being taken to reduce their on-call duties. The week is five days long for a start and is likely to include one night first on call for emergency admissions and one second on call. When first on call the houseman may be up for most of the night, but this currently gives no dispensation from the next day's work. One half day is supposed to be free for study or relaxation. One weekend in three the houseman lives in on first or second call. Two weeks' holiday are allowed in each six month post together with additional days for bank holidays worked. Radical improvement in both working conditions and educational opportunities of house officers are long overdue and the UK deans are working hard to achieve it.

When two house jobs have been completed satisfactorily, as they almost invariably are, the first period of a doctor's training is complete and he or she can apply for registration with the General Medical Council. Now the first career decisions must be made.

Choosing a specialty

I don't see being a doctor as a job — I see it as a way of life.
DAWN ADAMSON (1994)

... adjustments in the profession must be inevitable: when the adjustments are made it is essential that they do not continue to disadvantage those (men as well as women) who recognise their need for, and responsibility to, personal partners and children.
YVONNE NOBEL (1993)

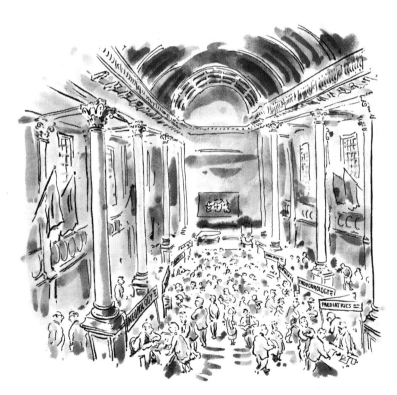

Before deciding finally whether to learn medicine, it is worth taking stock of the constraints that becoming a doctor will impose on family commitments or other interests, especially in the early postgraduate years. Not only the parent or the carer of elderly

Choosing a specialty

relatives but also the dedicated sportsman, musician, or enthusiast for a full life may have legitimate concerns about whether the job, a job they will very likely enjoy, would unacceptably monopolise their lives and stifle their interests. Given the structure of society and the traditionally predominant responsibility of mother for the family, many of the issues particularly concern women in medicine.

The largely inevitable but soluble conflict between the roles of mother and doctor arises from long hours, resident on-call duties, and new shift arrangements designed to reduce hours but creating their own problems in turn, both for structured life and for systematic postgraduate education. Doctors in accident and emergency departments usually work a round-the-clock shift system. Some other departments are beginning to work a partial shift system with several weeks on days interspersed with a week on night duty. Other departments are forming larger teams to reduce the night and weekend on-call duties of an otherwise traditional rota system. The maximum permitted average contracted hours of duty for doctors in training has recently fallen to 83 hours a week. Further reduction to 72 hours by the end of 1994 will be very difficult to achieve without substantially reducing the continuity of care of patients and giving the doctors on-call at night an extremely large number of patients to cover, most of whom will be unknown to them. One way or another (and there are several possible ways) the government is determined to achieve the target.

Provided both partners are prepared to share fully the tasks of house and home, postgraduate medical education can be combined with domestic commitments. The trouble is that more than 50% of married doctors are themselves married to doctors, with all the difficulty that entails, for coordinating on-call duties, for finding geographically convenient higher specialist training programmes, and eventually obtaining mutually compatible career posts. There may simply not be two appropriate posts in reasonably accessible locations within a reasonable time. If both partners are in the same specialty the possibility of job sharing initially might arise until a second post became available, but that proposition might neither please the employing authority nor satisfy the doctors themselves. General practice is a better bet in this regard, not least because home and practice are frequently close together. One couple, for example, took over a single-handed country practice and successfully shared both the practice and the home duties. Their patients, who had continuity of care from a close-knit partnership, benefited enormously while their children had the full attention of both their parents.

Women are as capable as men of success in any specialty in medicine. It is not clear why women are less well represented in some specialties than in others: do some specialties appeal more to men than women and vice versa? Is the difference related to some specialties being more demanding in their unsocial hours? Or is it the outcome of continued male prejudice in some specialties? The answer is perhaps a mixture of the first two but, today, very little of the last. Women tend to choose medical specialties in preference to surgical, with the exception of ophthalmology, but if they choose surgery they are not at a disadvantage. Paediatrics and public health are the only two specialties initially chosen by women more frequently than men.

Both men and women doctors take time to arrive at their final choice of specialty. Towards the end of the preregistration period, choices for paediatrics, general medicine, general surgery and obstetrics and gynaecology exceed opportunity. Preferences for pathology and radiology are about matched to opportunity, and psychiatry, general practice, and public health are undersubscribed. Over the next few years 25–33% of doctors change their choice, some more than once. About 40% of the changes of preference (and of 60% of women with children) are because of family commitments. Some specialties are more readily compatible with other responsibilities, such as general practice, both in its flexibility of working practice and in the earlier attainment of a settled home and secure income. Hospital specialities, which allow other commitments through well organised duty rotas, or light on-call responsibility, or by providing part-time work, include anaesthetics, accident and emergency, psychiatry, pathology, radiology, oncology and medicine for the elderly. Public health offers regular and reasonable hours. Overall, a recent survey showed that 50% of women and 25% of men considered marriage to have been a constraint on their career in medicine. But at the end of the day a final and realistic decision has to be made, balancing ambitions against the practicalities of personal responsibilities and professional training. In this, medicine is by no means unique.

A determined effort is being made to introduce good opportunities for "flexible training" but more still needs to be done to reduce the conflict between marriage and career in medicine and to diminish the relatively greater disadvantage of women. Practical measures needed include widespread provision of creches in the NHS and a means, perhaps through tax allowance, of offsetting the costs of assistance with child care. Better career advice is needed, both at medical school and in the early postgraduate years, together with more flexible training programmes. Most of this is happening, but too slowly. Most doctors do, eventually, find their way through the maze, but they and their families deserve more signposts and smoother paths.

Choosing a specialty

Several provisions have been made to help women retain professional involvement through years of heavy family responsibility. These are a step, but only a small step, in the right direction. A retainer scheme for married women provides an opportunity for them to undertake some specially arranged clinical sessions and to attend postgraduate teaching sessions; a small retainer fee is paid towards expenses such as registration with the General Medical Council, subscription to a medical defence organisation (insurance against claims for professional liability), and subscription to a recognised professional journal. When the doctor has more time a part time supernumerary training post may be created in the specialty of choice at a convenient hospital; the operative word is "may" because considerations of national career prospects in that specialty, of finance, and of daunting bureaucracy may well delay a decision for a year or more. A small proportion of established (not supernumerary) specialties has now been earmarked for part-time training.

PURSUING SPECIALIST TRAINING

A specialty needs to be chosen within two or three years of graduation and sights set on an appropriate route to a permanent career post. Most students qualify with little idea of the wide range of career opportunities open to them, an ignorance which reflects badly both on medical schools for not opening their students' eyes and on students for being so remarkably lacking in curiosity about their own future.

Careers fairs are held annually in several parts of the country to display the attractions of different specialites and to offer advice from doctors in all major specialties on a personal and informal level. Advice is available in medical schools from postgraduate subdeans, and in each district general hospital from the clinical tutor. Each region of the National Health Service also has a regional postgraduate dean, who is responsible for coordinating postgraduate training and advising individuals, mainly through the clinical tutors. Each royal college also has nominated regional advisers to whom trainees can turn.

Career decisions depend on many factors but a clear idea of the very wide opportunities available is the first necessity. Professional preference is only one consideration, a consideration all too often conditioned by the fact that most teachers of clinical medicine are general physicians and general surgeons, who, wittingly or unwittingly, give the impression that these are the only two worthy careers. House officer posts are also more or less confined to these specialties.

Choosing a specialty

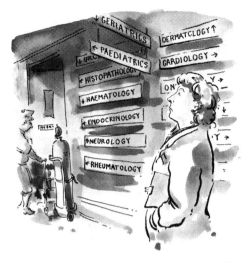

The major initial career preference is between clinical practice on the one hand and clinical support services on the other. Clinical practice may be in hospital or outside, mostly in general practice. Within hospital the clinical services broadly divide between those which are surgically based and those which are not. Clinical support services in hospital fall into two groups, laboratory based investigations and imaging based investigations. Support services outside hospital are broadly concerned with the framework of health of populations rather than of individuals, in short with public health. Some fortunate people decide on their careers as students ("fortunate" if they have made a realistic decision), more decide as housemen, and most decide in the next year or two while undertaking general professional training in senior house officer posts. Most senior house officer posts are not part of a specialist training programme but offer general training and experience. They are vital feet finding posts. *Living Medicine*, my sequel to this book, outlines the career options and specialty requirements in some detail (see Appendix 3).

MARKET FORCES

For years too many doctors have wanted to specialise in hospital specialties such as general medicine and general surgery and too few in, for example, pathology, psychiatry, geriatrics, and mental handicap. Most doctors, whether deciding to work in or out of hospital, have also wanted to live in green pastures, not in inner cities. A large number of doctors now choose general practice as their first choice. Many see general practice as more compatible than hospital specialties with a life of their own.

Choosing a specialty

Although a consultant post is the usual goal of a doctor working in hospital, there are career posts in the associate specialist grade which carry less responsibility. Many doctors, most of them general practitioners, also work part time in hospital on a sessional basis as clinical assistants or hospital practitioners.

Doctors are not in short supply overall, only selectively in some less popular specialties and in large cities. Sooner or later human resources will catch up with the need, if only because posts will become increasingly hard to find as the output of the medical schools increases. In the words of George Bernard Shaw, "Up to a certain point doctors, like carpenters and masons, must earn their living by doing work that the public wants from them."

EXPECTATION AND REALITY

It is necessary to be prepared for a gap between expectations of public admiration, respect, and gratitude and the often harder reality. Dr David Bradford, writing to encourage a young doctor who recently published a very dispirited account of her disillusionment in the *British Medical Journal*, eloquently described the reality and the compensation:

"I too found the practice of medicine vastly different from the theory. Patients were often messy, dirty, irresponsible, non-compliant, disagreeable, and self indulgent to the detriment of their health ... But medicine has a knack of working its healing touch on patients and practitioners alike. The more I looked after people in all their general untidiness the more I began to see the specks of gold in all of them."

Career opportunities

Surgery is superior to Medicine, because among other things it is
more lucrative. To receive gifts or money, a surgeon dare not fear
stench, must be able to cut like an executioner, politely lie and be
clever ... The sick above all want to be cured; the surgeon to be paid.
HENRI DE MONDEVILLE (thirteenth century)

The Royal Colleges are, of course, much the smarter end of the
profession; they represent the big time. However, the two main
Colleges, the Physicians and the Surgeons, are very different in
character. The Royal College of Physicians, like the Catholic Church,
is ancient and obscurely hierarchical. It occupies a tiny Vatican in
Regents Park, whose benign soft-footed cardinals pad around discussing preferment of one kind or another. To be a Member of the
College (achieved by examination) counts for nothing at all. One must
be elected a Fellow. ... In turning to the College of Surgeons one
moves from the episcopal to the military. Surgeons are brash,
extrovert characters who pride themselves on energy rather than
subtlety. Fellowship is decided by examination, and theoretically all
Fellows are equal, just as theoretically all officers are gentlemen.
JOHN ROWAN WILSON (1972)

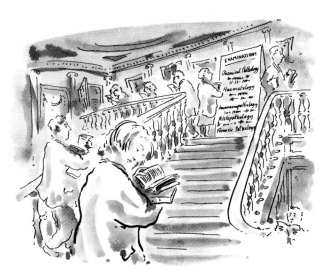

Notwithstanding the traditional polarisation of medicine and surgery, most graduates become neither a consultant physician nor a
consultant surgeon. About half the graduates of medical schools in

Career opportunities

the United Kingdom become general practitioners, a quarter become hospital consultants, and an eighth become specialists working in the community either in public health or in community health clinical work. This chapter deals with the major higher professional qualifications (table IV) and the range of career posts for which these qualifications are required (table V).

TABLE IV—*Major professional higher qualifications*

Diploma	Full title
MRCP*	Membership of the Royal Colleges of Physicians of the United Kingdom
FRCS	Fellowship of the Royal College of Surgeons
FCA	Fellowship of the College of Anaesthetists
MRCOG*	Membership of the Royal College of Obstetricians and Gynaecologists
MRCPsych*	Membership of the Royal College of Psychiatrists
MRCPath*	Membership of the Royal College of Pathologists
FRCR	Fellowship of the Royal College of Radiologists
MRCGP*	Membership of the Royal College of General Practitioners
MPHM*	Membership of the Faculty of Public Health Medicine of the Royal College of Physicians

*Fellowship is by election after an interval of several years.

Accreditation as a specialist is given when the required training programme is completed, but that does not mean that a permanent career post is immediately available; the length of training and the difficulty in finding a career post vary with the specialty. A higher university degree such as an MD (doctor of medicine, awarded for a dissertation which is usually based on clinical research undertaken in the course of postgraduate training) or a PhD (doctor of philosophy, awarded for a thesis based on two or three years of supervised, whole time laboratory research) is a useful and sometimes essential additional qualification.

All specialist training programmes begin after two preregistration house officer posts and a year or two of general training and experience in senior house officer posts in hospital (general professional training). Sometimes the general training is undertaken overseas or in the armed services on a short service commission. A year as a registrar in some specialties is also suitable general professional training.

GENERAL PRACTICE

To be eligible to become an assistant or a principal in general practice a doctor must complete three years' vocational training. This includes at least 12 months as a trainee general practitioner, two periods of at least six months each in educationally approved training posts drawn from a list of hospital specialties particularly relevant to general practice, such as paediatrics, geriatrics, obstetrics, psychiatry, and accident and emergency, and the remainder

Career opportunities

TABLE V—*Major specialties and their required professional higher qualifications*

Specialty	Qualification
General practice	MRCGP†
Hospital specialties	
Accident and emergency*	FRCS, MRCP, FCA, or MRCGP
Anaesthesia	FCA
Medicine:	MRCP
General (internal) medicine	
Paediatrics	
Cardiology	
Clinical immunology (see also pathology)	
Clinical pharmacology	
Communicable (infectious) diseases	
Dermatology*	
Endocrinology and diabetes	
Genitourinary medicine (venereology)*	
Geriatrics*	
Haematology (see also pathology)*	
Neurology	
Oncology (see also radiotherapy)	
Renal disease (nephrology)	
Respiratory disease	
Rheumatology*	
Tropical medicine	
Obstetrics and gynaecology	MRCOG
Pathology:*	MRCPath
Clinical biochemistry	
Haematology	
Blood transfusion	
Histopathology	
Immunopathology	
Medical microbiology	
Forensic pathology	
Clinical immunology	

of the time in hospital or community medicine (fig 1). Any or all of the training may be undertaken part time provided the whole training is completed within seven years.

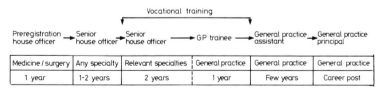

General practitioners are still in short supply in some parts of the country, and any suitably qualified doctor may set up a practice in those areas for the asking. In other areas a vacancy created by retirement must be awaited. Unfortunately the structure of employment of general practitioners counts doctors' heads and not the number of patients served: in some inner city areas there are

89

Career opportunities

Table V continued

Specialty	Qualification
Psychiatry:*	MRCPsych
Child psychiatry	
Forensic psychiatry	
Mental handicap	
Psychogeriatrics	
Psychotherapy	
Diagnostic radiology*	FRCR
Radiotherapy and oncology*	FRCR (MRCP)
Surgery:	FRCS
General surgery	
Neurosurgery	
Orthopaedics	
Otorhinolaryngology	
Ophthalmology	FCO
Paediatric surgery	
Plastic surgery	
Urology	
*Public health medicine**	MPHM
Other specialties	
Occupational medicine*	MRCP, MFOM
Armed services	
Pharmaceutical industry*	
Full time research	
Basic medical sciences*	
Medical journalism*	

*Relatively more suitable for part time training and employment.
†MRCGP is not essential for entry to general practice.

many doctors but, because many keep their lists of National Health Service patients small to enable them to take on other medical work, patients may find a doctor hard to get. The need for more doctors exists, but they are not permitted to come in to meet that need. Vacancies are advertised and filled in open competition. It is usual now to move directly into a partnership rather than serving as an assistant in a practice first.

General practice is a demanding but fulfilling career. One attraction is the prospect of a settled home and higher income at an early stage than a career in the hospital service. If you also live in the district in which you practise you naturally become very much part of the community in which you live. Part time posts in general practice convenient for doctors who want or need to give part of their time to other responsibilities are not too difficult to find.

After completing a three year training scheme or after being fully registered for four years, of which two have been spent in general practice, a doctor may take the examination for membership of the Royal College of General Practitioners (MRCGP), but it is not an essential qualification.

Career opportunities

The formal training for most hospital specialties takes about six years after general professional training (fig 2), making a total of about eight after full registration before specialist accreditation is received, but this is about to be shortened in line with training in other countries of the European Community by about two years. In relatively undersubscribed specialties, such as radiology, histopathology, chemical pathology, medical microbiology, geriatrics, psychiatry, and mental handicap, a permanent career post may be obtained before the formal training is finished, whereupon de facto accreditation as a specialist is given. In oversubscribed specialties, such as general medicine, paediatrics, and general surgery, a permanent post may not be secured until a few years after accreditation. Attempts are now being made to limit entry to specialties to the number of doctors who can expect to secure a career post within a short time of completing their formal training. Posts of senior house officer and above are advertised nationally and filled in open competition.

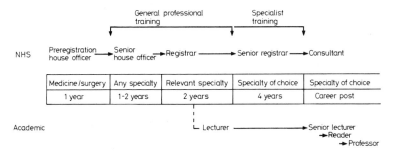

FIG 2—Structure of training for a hospital specialty in either the National Health Service or clinical academic posts (but see note above).

Although the broad pattern of specialty training is similar in hospital based specialities the nature of the work and the higher qualifications required are quite different. Some specialties, such as general medicine, general surgery, and obstetrics and gynaecology, involve substantial resident duties at nights and weekends (and are correspondingly better paid at junior level though not at consultant level because consultants do not receive extra duty payments), while others, such as most pathology specialties, offer regular hours and light on call duties.

A progression from registrar through senior registrar to consultant looks tidy and simple and would be were it not for the fact that in the most popular specialties registrar posts substantially outnumber senior registrar posts (which are held for longer) and in some specialties the number of consultant posts expected to become vacant is too small for the number of senior registrars in training. New proposals would merge the registrar and senior registrar into a single training grade and shorten the period of training.

The reasons why organisation of an efficient career structure in hospital specialties has proved too difficult for the experts are many and complex. Steps are being taken to rationalise the structure, but progress will be slow and threatens to change the nature of consultant posts. None the less, change there has to be to prevent years of training being wasted by failure to navigate the bottleneck between registrar and senior registrar, and to prevent the frustration caused to those who have satisfactorily completed their training only to find no opportunity to achieve independence. Whatever happens it is clear that would-be specialists in hospital will need to continue to be flexible in moving anywhere in the country where opportunity lies both for training and for a career post. When husband and wife are each pursuing a professional career this need to seek one's fortune may cause many problems. Improvement in the career structure for doctors should result before long in a better opportunity for an individual to obtain most, if not all, training in one part of the country to avoid the domestic disruption caused by a series of uncoordinated training posts.

Accident and emergency

It is both odd and sad that this front line of the hospital service used to be a Cinderella specialty, but this is now changing rapidly. Departments have in the past been managed part time by an orthopaedic surgeon or other member of staff who has other major responsibilities. Career training posts have been few. Part of the problem has been that patients tend to use hospital accident and emergency departments as a short cut to general practitioner services. On the one hand, the real accidents and emergencies become submerged (and the doctors with them) and, on the other hand, the patient receives less than optimum service, partly because of the lack of continuity of care.

General practice is much better provided by general practitioners than by hospitals, but in inner cities much of the task of providing primary health care falls on accident and emergency departments because general practitioner services are often not readily available. At the same time there is a large floating population which does not even attempt to register with a general practitioner. The nature of the work in an accident and emergency department is so wide that a higher qualification in either surgery, medicine, anaesthetics, or general practice is acceptable for the consultant in charge.

Anaesthesia

Anaesthetists belong to a College of Anaesthetists. Providing pain relief or anaesthesia during surgical operations, childbirth, and diagnostic procedures is their major task, but they often also take a special interest in the intensive care of critically ill patients. Anaesthesia is a large and expanding specialty. Emergency duties are heavy, but as anaesthetists do not normally have continuing responsibility for patients it is possible to structure a shift system in duty rotas. Part time sessional appointments in anaesthesia are available in the clinical assistant grade.

The primary examination for fellowship of the College of Anaesthetists (FCA) is usually taken during a senior house officer post in anaesthesia and is a test of knowledge of the scientific basis of anaesthesia. The final part of the FCA is taken at least three years after full registration and after two years in approved anaesthetic posts. Higher training is undertaken as a senior registrar once the FCA has been obtained and lasts three years, one of which may be spent in research.

Medicine

Medicine covers a large area of hospital work. By far the largest specialty within it is general (internal) medicine. It sounds paradoxical to have a general specialty, but, unlike the task of a general practitioner, more or less all the work of a general physician is medical, whereas a general practitioner must have a good working knowledge of the preliminary diagnosis and treatment of all common conditions whether medical, surgical, psychiatric, gynaecological, or obstetric. General physicians usually have special interest and experience in one particular subspecialty; some physicians become superspecialists and confine all their work to one discipline such as cardiology or rheumatology.

"Internal" is added to the title of general medicine because that is the North American term for the specialty. Most British hospitals are not large enough to have a superspecialist in each subspecialty of medicine, and for that reason alone an adequate service cannot be provided if the consultant physicians are too specialised. Furthermore, the physicians spend much of their time dealing with general medical emergencies, which not only demand competence over a wide field of medicine but overlap with surgical emergencies. Another reason for specialists in medicine remaining competent over a wide field is that it simply is not possible to be sure with most patients at an early state of diagnosis which superspecialist (if any) would be most appropriate to undertake further investigation and treatment.

Time and again a good general opinion is needed rather than intensely specialised knowledge. This is reflected in the story told by the late Professor J R A Mitchell of Nottingham of a patient who reappeared in the professor's outpatient clinic having been tossed from specialist to specialist saying: "There is no point sending me to another specialist, doctor. It's not my special parts which have gone wrong but what holds them together."

Membership of the Royal Colleges of Physicians of the United Kingdom (MRCP(UK)) is the professional diploma needed before embarking on specialist training in any of the specialties listed under medicine in table V. There are royal colleges in London, Edinburgh, and Glasgow but they now hold a common membership examination. Election to fellowship of one of these colleges follows about 10 years after the member has passed the examination for membership, depending on friends, influence, distinction, or a subtle mixture of all three.

The MRCP diploma is a necessary entry qualification but confers no right to training in a medical specialty. More doctors are successful in the examination than can become specialists in medicine. Some deliberately acquire the diplomas as an additional qualification before entering another hospital specialty or general practice. Part I of the examination can be taken 18 months after graduation and comprises mutliple choice questions covering a wide range of medicine and the sciences immediately relevant to it. Part II consists of a written section with questions on case histories and slides, a searching clinical examination, and an oral examination. The clinical and oral examinations are taken either in adult medicine or paediatrics.

The MRCP examination is above all a test of clinical skills. In principle it tests the same as the final MB examination but at a more demanding and discriminating level. It is necessary to know about rarities but it is also essential to have sound clinical common sense.

Obstetrics and gynaecology

Obstetrics and gynaecology form one specialty. Obstetrics offers a balance between medicine and surgery with the attraction of usually young and healthy patients. Gynaecology also demands both surgical and medical skills together with a substantial amount of human understanding.

Specialists in this field need to become members of the Royal College of Obstetricians and Gynaecologists (MRCOG). Part I of the examination, a multiple choice paper on the basic sciences related to the specialty, may be taken at any time after full registration. Part II is taken after at least three years in approved posts and includes written, clinical, and oral examinations together with preparation of case records and commentaries. Instruction in family planning is included in the training. Many obstetricians train first in general surgery and obtain the Fellowship of the Royal College of Surgeons (FRCS) to acquire a much wider surgical expertise than their limited field demands, and a few start in medicine and pass the MRCP. An occasional brilliant workhorse obtains both these diplomas and the MRCOG.

Pathology

The specialties of pathology provide a wide range of laboratory diagnostic services, which are an essential part of everyday clinical practice. The clinical biochemist is an expert in the biochemical diagnosis of disease; the histopathologist an expert in diagnosing disease from changes in tissue structure; and the medical microbiologist (a title which includes bacteriologist, virologist, and mycologist) an expert in the culture and identification of bacteria, viruses, fungi, and other communicable causes of disease. The haematologist is concerned with disorders of the blood and with blood transfusion; some haematologists specialise entirely in blood transfusion and work for the National Blood Transfusion Service. Clinical immunology is a small but expanding specialty which spans laboratory science and clinical medicine; it is concerned particularly with the role of immune reactions in disease.

Although based in the laboratory, pathologists often consult on patients at their colleagues' request. The medical microbiologist, for example, should be in a position to give expert advice on antibiotic treatment of difficult infections. Haematologists normally have patients under their care in wards and outpatients. Besides having scientific and clinical skills the consultant pathologist needs to be a good organiser of a laboratory and its staff.

For a career in all these pathology specialties (with the exception of clinical immunology, for which the MRCP may be more appropriate) it is necessary to become a member of the Royal College of Pathologists (MRCPath). The part I examination is taken after at least two years in recognised training posts and tests knowledge of all branches of pathology. Part II is taken after at least three further years of experience in one branch of pathology, and the examination is limited to that branch. Unlike the MRCP, which is in effect an entry qualification to specialisation in medicine, acquisition of the MRCPath marks the completion of training as a pathologist.

Career opportunities

Psychiatry

Psychiatry is an expanding specialty which is changing rapidly, not least because new treatments are substantially reducing the need for inpatient treatment, especially the need for long stay mental hospitals. One of its most challenging subspecialties is mental handicap, a Cinderella subject with good job opportunities and immense potential for deploying a range of medical skills and human understanding to help the handicapped to realise their own abilities. Here too the emphasis is shifting from incarceration in large institutions to rehabilitation in a small unit before patients return to their own homes.

The examination for membership of the Royal College of Psychiatrists (MRCPsych) may be taken after three years of approved experience, most of which has to be in psychiatry. This means working as a registrar and senior registrar in a psychiatric hospital looking after both emergency and long stay patients besides seeing patients in the psychiatric outpatient clinic. It is possible to specialise in either adult or child psychiatry, but all psychiatrists will in future be expected to have some experience of both.

A good knowledge of medicine is valuable to psychiatry, and psychiatrists often acquire the MRCP in the early years of their training. Although psychiatry is clearly one important aspect of the management of mental handicap, the subject demands wider skills.

Diagnostic radiology

Like pathologists, radiologists need to be good organisers because sooner or later they will have to organise a department. They need to be good with their hands in performing investigative techniques, such as angiography, and sharp with their eyes and brains in interpreting films. Many radiologists obtain the MRCP or, occasionally, the FRCS while gaining wide clinical experience before taking up radiology. Diagnostic radiology serves all clinical departments and often provides a service for general practitioners as well. The radiologist therefore has a natural link with most of his colleagues. Radiologists have contact with patients without clinical responsibility for their treatment; out of hours duties are not heavy.

Fellowship of the Royal College of Radiologists (FRCR) is a necessary qualification. Part I is taken after at least one year in a recognised training post as registrar and part II after at least three years of training as a registrar then senior registrar.

Career opportunities

Radiotherapy and oncology

Cancer is treated by radiotherapy, drugs, or surgery or by a combination of these approaches. Treatment of cancer entirely or partly by irradiation (radiotherapy), or entirely by drugs (chemotherapy) is usually organised by different individuals, the clinical oncologist (sometimes still called radiotherapist), and the medical oncologist, respectively. They undertake overlapping but partly different training, are expected to obtain the FRCR (and may obtain the MRCP also), and they often work in close collaboration. Successful treatment of cancer requires teamwork, and clinical oncologists and medical oncologists work closely with colleagues in other specialties, especially with surgeons, physicians, and gynaecologists.

Part I of the FRCR examination is common to diagnostic radiology and radiotherapy but they have a different Part II examination.

Surgery

Surgical training is now divided into two parts: basic surgical training applicable to those in all surgical specialties, and higher surgical training in which the surgeon decides on the specialty that he or she is going to pursue and continues training in that area only.

Basic surgical training follows house officer appointments and lasts for two years. At the end of that time the trainee should have sufficient knowledge and skills to pursue further training in the surgical specialty of his or her choice. Basic training includes the basic sciences, general surgery, accident and emergency, and orthopaedic surgery. There is an examination at the conclusion of this period, which is currently known as the FRCS, although it may possibly change its title.

The trainee then enrols in higher surgical training. This takes five or six years and at present is divided into registrar and senior registrar, although these two grades will shortly be amalgamated into a continuum of training. There are eight recognised specialties, one of which is general surgery; the others include, for example, surgery, plastic surgery, and urology. Towards the end of this period of higher surgical training, there is a further examination in that specialty which is an Intercollegiate Examination run by the four surgical colleges of Great Britain and Ireland.

PUBLIC HEALTH MEDICINE

Public health is the medical speciality which is concerned to improve the health of populations — by health promotion, by disease prevention, and by the delivery of high quality, value for money health care. Public health doctors work closely with doctors

97

100 DOCTORS

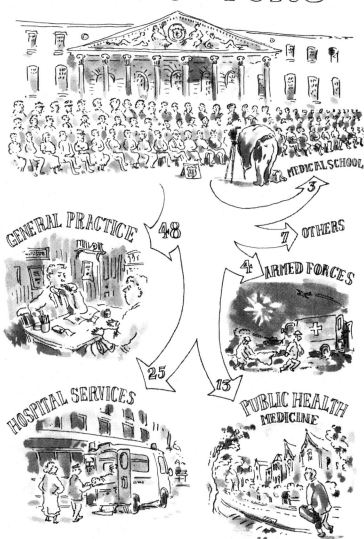

in many specialties, and with other health professionals, with managers, and with governmental and voluntary organisations in achieving their aims.

Public health recognises that health requires more than individual patient care. If all members of society are to achieve a better and more equitable health status and health experience, collective action is essential.

Epidemiology is the science fundamental to public health medicine with important contributions from statistics and social sciences. Public health practitioners also require a range of other skills, most crucially those associated with management, interpersonal, and political skills.

Public health physicians work in a number of settings within the NHS, academic departments, and central government and national agencies such as the Health Education Authority and the Communicable Disease Surveillance Centre.

Two years of general professional and early specialist training culminate in Part I of the examination for Membership of the Faculty of Public Health Medicine (MFPHM) of the Royal Colleges of Physicians, which covers epidemiology, statistics, social and behavioural sciences, the principles of prevention of disease and promotion of health, assessment of health needs, and audit of services provided, environmental health, and the management and organisation of health services. It is a rapidly expanding field. During three years of higher specialist training, the trainee in public health medicine writes a report on practical projects as part of the requirement for Part II of the MFPHM examination.

COMMUNITY HEALTH

Doctors working in community health are clinical specialists providing a wide range of services including child health, family planning, mental and physical handicap, genetic counselling, occupational, environmental and port health, and services for the elderly. The relevant clinical specialist training, or GP vocational training, is the usual qualification for this work, but there are as yet no formal, relevant, community, higher specialist training programmes or qualifications.

The future of the grades of clinical medical officer (CMO) and senior clinical medical officer (SCMO) is uncertain; these are career posts without time limits under the terms and conditions of service for doctors working in public health medicine and community health which often offer opportunities for long term, part time employment. There are a small but increasing number of consultant posts in these community specialities, and training programmes for these posts are being developed.

OTHER SPECIALTIES

Occupational medicine—Occupational medicine is a recently developed clinical specialty which includes the former discipline of industrial medicine. The specialty is concerned with identifying and investigating the medical problems of work and with advising both management and employees on the prevention of medical hazards of occupations. The examination for membership of the Faculty of Occupational Medicine (MFOM) of the Royal College of Physicians is taken after four years of training and experience in occupational medicine, but there is not yet a formal higher specialist training programme.

Armed services—The three major branches of the armed services offer careers for both specialists and general practitioners on long or short term contracts. Many doctors begin a service career with a short service commission while they are medical students. In return for a good salary during clinical training and the preregistration year these doctors are required to serve for a further five years in the armed services.

Pharmaceutical industry—The pharmaceutical industry is employing an increasing number of doctors in clinical research and in an advisory capacity. Most doctors entering the industry have a good background in clinical pharmacology or medicine.

Full time research—The small number of full time research posts available to medical graduates are mainly in institutions of the Medical Research Council or the pharmaceutical industry.

Clinical academic medicine—An academic career is possible in practically all hospital specialties, general practice, and community medicine, though the number of posts is small. Senior lecturers, readers, and professors all normally have consultant responsibilities, but they have less clinical service work and relatively more time than Health Service consultants for teaching and research.

Basic medical sciences—It is widely but not universally believed that medical students benefit from being taught anatomy, physiology, biochemistry, and pharmacology from medical graduates working in these subjects, mainly because they are in the best position to judge the relevance of science to its application in clinical medicine. The salaries of medical graduates working in preclinical departments are lower than those of clinical academics or of doctors working in the National Health Service.

Medical journalism—Few opportunities exist for full time posts in medical journalism, but the *British Medical Journal*, *The Lancet*, and a number of other publications have full time medically qualified editors (and some who are not medically qualified). Many specialist medical journals have part time medical editors, as do several newspapers and industrially sponsored medical publications. Freelance opportunities abound for doctors with lively minds and ready pens.

Postscript

In remembering those with whom I was year after year associated,
and whom it was my duty to study, nothing appears more certain than
that the personal character, the very nature, the will of each student
had far greater force in determining his career than any helps or
hindrances whatever.

SIR JAMES PAGET (1869)

Growing as a person means coming to recognise and accept the follies
and frailties of our own humanity. And for this I believe that there is
no greater teacher than the practice of medicine.

DAVID BRADFORD (1993)

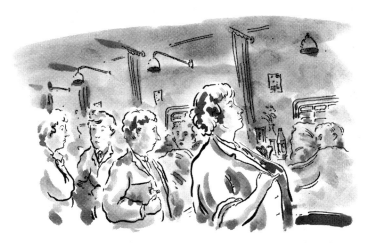

There is no royal road to learning medicine. The path is long, the
demands heavy, and the sacrifices real. Learning never stops: it
starts when the student is a spectator but sinks deep only when
learning is through service. All doctors must continue to learn, and
not only about new advances but to appreciate the limitations of all
knowledge. They also need to learn humility in the face of their
own imperfect understanding and their patients' courage.

Hard though the road may be, the satisfaction at the end of it is
in danger of being underplayed, not least by the rather dishearten-
ing note on which the BBC television series *Doctors To Be* ended.

101

Postscript

In contrast, a recent graduate, who had more than her fair share of difficulties during the course, wrote recently:

> "I am now working in a friendly but busy district general hospital and I love it. I love being a doctor. I hate some of it, but I am glad I went through medical school, resits and all!"

Although medicine is learnt to be practised it would be a poor academic discipline if it were not an education in itself. The academic study of medicine can fulfil the broader objectives of a university education as well as any other subject, objectives which have never been better expressed than by the late E A Welbourne, one time master of Emmanuel College, Cambridge:

> We are content to see men (and women) turn into themselves and admit to themselves their abilities and their limitations. We hope that they leave us with some understanding of the nature of knowledge and memorised formulae, with some experience of the nature of understanding and its difference from the acceptance of authority and, still more, from rejection of authority through even greater, if similar, credulity; with some ability to reach agreement, at first with their friends, and as time passes with others, and to understand that argument and explanation is not for victory but to reach agreement. We hope that they will be able to resist the stream of propaganda in a world deluged with progaganda. ... We hope that they will have been encouraged in honesty and stoutness of heart ...

At the end of the day, however, it may well be that the hallmark of a competent doctor is, in the words of the late Sir George Pickering, lately regius professor of medicine at Oxford, "that he knows what he can do and what he cannot do. The best doctors know to whom to turn for help."

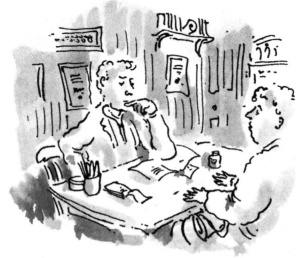

Appendix 1:
Goals and objectives of undergraduate medical education

(a) The student should acquire a *knowledge* and *understanding* of health and its promotion, and of disease, its prevention, and management, in the context of the whole individual and his or her place in the family and in society.
(b) The student should acquire and become proficient in basic clinical *skills*, such as the ability to obtain a patient's history, to undertake a comprehensive physical and mental state examination and interpret the findings, and to demonstrate competence in the performance of a limited number of basic technical procedures.
(c) The student should acquire and demonstrate *attitudes* necessary for the achievement of high standards of medical practice, both in relation to the provision of care of individuals and populations, and to his or her own personal development.

OBJECTIVES
Knowledge objectives

At the end of the undergraduate course the student will have acquired a knowledge and understanding of:

(a) The *sciences basic to medicine*, and
    (i) the discovery of how knowledge is acquired;
    (ii) an understanding of research methods;
    (iii) an ability to evaluate evidence.
(b) The *range of problems* that are presented to doctors and the *range of solutions* that have been developed for their recognition, investigation, prevention, and treatment.
(c) *Diseases* in terms of *processes*, both mental and physical, such as trauma, inflammation, immune response, degeneration, neoplasia, metabolic disturbance, and genetic disorder.
(d) How *disease presents* in patients of all ages, how patients react to illness or to the belief that they are ill, and how illness behaviour varies among social and cultural groups.
(e) The *environmental* and *social determinants* of disease, the principles of disease surveillance and the means by which diseases may spread, and the analysis of the burden of disease within the community.
(f) The principles of *disease prevention* and *health promotion*.
(g) The principles of *therapy*, including:
    (i) the management of acute illness;
    (ii) the actions of drugs, their prescription, and their administration;
    (iii) the care of the chronically ill and the disabled;
    (iv) rehabilitation, institutional, and community care;

(v) the amelioration of suffering and the relief of pain;

(vi) the care of the dying.

(h) *Reproduction*, including:

    (i) pregnancy and childbirth;

    (ii) fertility and contraception;

    (iii) psychological aspects.

(i) *Human relationships*, individual and community.

(j) The importance of *communication*, both with patients and their relatives and with other professionals, both medical and non-medical, involved in their care.

(k) Ethical and legal issues relevant to the practice of medicine.

(l) The *organisation, management,* and *provision of health care* both in the community and in hospital, the economic and practical constraints within which it is delivered, and the audit process to monitor its delivery.

Skills objectives

At the end of the course of undergraduate education the student will have acquired and demonstrated his or her proficiency in communication and the other essential skills of medicine, including:

(a) *Basic clinical method*, including the ability to:

    (i)   obtain and record a comprehensive history;

    (ii) perform a complete physical examination, and assess the mental state;

    (iii) interpret the findings obtained from the history and the physical examination;

    (iv) reach a provisional assessment of patients' problems and formulate with them plans for investigation and management.

(b) *Basic clinical procedures*, including:

    (i)   basic and advanced life support;

    (ii) venepuncture;

    (iii) insertion of an intravenous line.

[This is a restricted list. Doctors undertaking procedures on patients must at all stages in their careers be fully competent in their performance or be under the close supervision of those so competent. Patients are entitled to expect no less and those employing doctors must have confidence in the adequacy of their training. If practical skills are allowed to lapse they should be reacquired, again under supervision. There is a limit to the number and type of procedures that it is proper for students to undertake on patients, and witnessing or assisting at their performance by others should not be assumed to endow a significant level of competence. The appropriate time for the acquisition of most of the basic practical skills is during the preregistration year when educational supervisors have responsibility for ensuring the adequacy of training.

The information available to the Education Committee indicates that schools can identify the range of procedures undertaken by their students, but we now recommend that they construct a list of those procedures in each of which they will require all students to have demonstrated competence by the time that they qualify. This list, which should be compiled in consultation with Postgraduate Deans and higher training bodies, should be known not only to students and their teachers but also to preregistration house officers, educational supervisors, and employers.]

(c) Basic computing skills as applied to medicine.

Attitudinal objectives

At the end of the course of undergraduate medical education the student will have acquired and will demonstrate attitudes essential to the practice of medicine, including:

(a) Respect for patients and colleagues that encompasses, without prejudice, diversity of background and opportunity, language, culture, and way of life.

(b) The recognition of patients' rights in all respects, and particularly in regard to confidentiality and informed consent.

(c) Approaches to learning that are based on curiosity and the exploration of knowledge rather than on its passive acquisition, and that will be retained throughout professional life.

(d) Ability to cope with uncertainty.

(e) Awareness of the moral and ethical responsibilities involved in individual patient care and in the provision of care to populations of patients: such awareness must be developed early in the course.

(f) Awareness of the need to ensure that the highest possible quality of patient care must always be provided.

(g) Development of capacity for self audit and for participation in the peer review process.

(h) Awareness of personal limitations, a willingness to seek help when necessary, and ability to work effectively as a member of a team.

(i) Willingness to use his or her professional capabilities to contribute to community as well as to individual patient welfare, by the practice of preventive medicine and the encouragement of health promotion.

(j) Ability to adapt to change.

(k) Awareness of the need for continuing professional development allied to the process of continuing medical education, to ensure that high levels of clinical competence and knowledge are maintained.

(l) Acceptance of the responsibility to contribute as far as possible to the advancement of medical knowledge for the benefit of medical practice and further improvement in the quality of patient care.

From *Tomorrow's Doctors—Recommendations on Undergraduate Medical Education*, General Medical Council, 1993.

Appendix 2:

Attributes of the independent practitioner

1 *The ability to solve clinical and other problems in medical practice* which involves or requires:

(a) an intellectual and temperamental ability to change, to face the unfamiliar, and to adapt to change;

  (b) a capacity for individual, self directed learning; and
  (c) reasoning and judgement in the application of knowledge to the analysis and interpretation of data, in defining the nature of a problem, and in planning and implementing a strategy to resolve it.

2 *Possession of adequate knowledge and understanding of the general structure and function of the human body and workings of the mind, in health and disease, of their interaction, and of the interaction between humans and their physical and social environment.* This requires:
  (a) knowledge of the physical, behavioural, epidemiological, and clinical sciences upon which medicine depends;
  (b) understanding of the aetiology and natural history of diseases;
  (c) understanding of the impact both of psychological factors upon illness and of illness upon the patient and the patient's family;
  (d) understanding the effects of childhood growth and of later ageing upon the individual, the family, and the community; and
  (e) understanding of the social, cultural, and environmental factors that contribute to health or illness, and the capacity of medicine to influence them.

3 *Possession of consultation skills,* which include:
  (a) skills in sensitive and effective communication with patients and their families, professional colleagues and local agencies, and the keeping of good medical records;
  (b) the clinical skills necessary to examine the patient's physical and mental state, and to investigate appropriately;
  (c) the ability to exercise sound clinical judgement to analyse symptoms and physical signs in pathophysiological terms, to establish diagnoses, and to offer advice to the patient taking account of physical, psychological, social, and cultural factors; and
  (d) understanding of the special needs of terminal care.

4 *Acquisition of a high standard of knowledge and skills in the doctor's specialty,* which include:
  (a) understanding of acute illness and of disabling and chronic diseases within that specialty, including their physical, mental, and social implications, rehabilitation, pain relief, and the need for support and encouragement; and
  (b) relevant manual, biochemical, pharmacological, psychological, social, and other interventions in acute and chronic illness.

5 *Willingness and ability to deal with common medical emergencies and with other illness in an emergency.*

6 *The ability to contribute appropriately to the prevention of illness and the promotion of health,* which involves:
  (a) understanding of the principles, methods, and limitations of preventive medicine and health promotion;
  (b) understanding of the doctor's role in educating patients, families, and communities, and in generally promoting good health; and
  (c) the ability to identify individuals at risk and to take appropriate action.

7 *The ability to recognise and analyse ethical problems so as to enable patients, their families, society, and the doctor to have proper regard to such problems in reaching decisions;* this comprehends:

(a) knowledge of the ethical standards and legal responsibilities of the medical profession;

(b) understanding of the impact of medicosocial legislation of medical practice; and

(c) recognition of the influence upon his or her approach to ethical problems of the doctor's own personality and values.

8 *The maintenance of attitudes and conduct appropriate to a high level of professional practice*, which includes:

(a) recognition that a blend of scientific and humanitarian approaches is required, involving a critical approach to learning, open-mindedness, compassion, and concern for the dignity of the patient and, where relevant, of the patient's family;

(b) recognition that good medical practice depends on partnership between doctor and patient, based upon mutual understanding and trust; the doctor may give advice, but the patient must decide whether or not to accept it;

(c) commitment to providing high quality care; awareness of the limitations of the doctor's own knowledge and of existing medical knowledge; recognition of the duty to keep up to date in the doctor's own specialist field and to be aware of developments in others; and

(d) willingness to accept review, including self audit, of the doctor's performance.

9 *Mastery of the skills required to work within a team and, where appropriate, assume the responsibilities of team leader*, which requires:

(a) recognition of the need for the doctor to collaborate in prevention, diagnosis, treatment, and management with other health care professionals and with patients themselves;

(b) understanding and appreciation of the roles, responsibilities, and skills of nurses and other health care workers; and

(c) the ability to lead, guide, and coordinate the work of others.

10 *Acquisition of experience in administration and planning*, including:

(a) efficient management of the doctor's own time and professional activities;

(b) appropriate use of diagnostic and therapeutic resources, and appreciation of the economic and practical constraints affecting the provision of health care; and

(c) willingness to participate, as required, in the work of bodies which advise, plan, and assist the development and administration of medical services, such as NHS authorities and trusts, Royal Colleges and Faculties, and professional associations.

11 *Recognition of the opportunities and acceptance of the duty to contribute, when possible, to the advancement of medical knowledge and skill*, which entails:

(a) understanding of the contribution of research methods, and interpretation and application of others' research in the doctor's own specialty; and

(b) willingness, when appropriate, to contribute to research in the doctor's specialist field, both personally and through encouraging participation by junior colleagues.

Appendices

12 *Recognition of the obligation to teach others, particularly doctors in training*, which requires:

   (a) acceptance of responsibility for training junior colleagues in the specialty, and for teaching other doctors, medical students, and other health care professionals, when required;

   (b) recognition that teaching skills are not necessarily innate but can be learned, and willingness to acquire them; and

   (c) recognition that the example of the teacher is the most powerful influence upon the standards of conduct and practice of every trainee.

From *Tomorrow's Doctors—Recommendations on Undergraduate Medical Education*, General Medical Council, 1993.

Appendix 3:
Suggestions for further reading

University and College Entrance: Official Guide 1995. London: UCAS 1994 (obtainable from Sheed & Ward Ltd, 14 Coopers Row, London EC3N 2BH). Price £12.00 plus £2.50 for postage and packing. An annual detailed list of all entry requirements.

A Doctor or Else? by J Thurman. 3rd ed. Norwich: Yare Valley Publishers, 1986.

How to Apply for Admission to a University. Cheltenham: Universities and Colleges Admission Service (PO Box 67, Cheltenham, Glos GL50 3SF). Yearly. An essential handbook revised annually with details on when and how to apply for medical school (and all other university courses).

Proper Doctoring by D Mendel. Berlin: Springer Verlag, 1984. (Obtainable from the author at Gilhams Cottage, Easterling, near Faversham, Kent ME13 0BP. Price £3.)

Invitation to Medicine by D A K Black. Oxford: Basil Blackwell, 1987. Price £4.95. Discusses the central features of contemporary medicine and the ways doctors work in practice.

Living Medicine: planning a career—choosing a speciality by Peter Richards. Cambridge: Cambridge University Press, 1990. Price £8.95. Carries on where *Learning Medicine* leaves off. Prepares those approaching Finals for the general responsibilities and specific opportunities of being a doctor.

Doctors To Be by Susan Spindler. London: BBC books, 1992. Price £12.95. The story of 10 medical students from selection to qualification and house jobs seen through the eyes of the producer of the BBC TV *Horizon* series "Doctors To Be".

Appendices
Appendix 4:
Addresses of medical schools

Medical School, University of Birmingham, Birmingham B15 2TJ.

Medical School, University of Bristol, Bristol BS8 1TH.

Medical School, University of Cambridge, Cambridge CB2 1TN.

School of Medicine, University of Leeds, Thoresby Place, Leeds LS2 9NL.

School of Medicine, University of Leicester, University Road, Leicester LE1 7RH.

Faculty of Medicine, University of Liverpool, PO Box 147, Liverpool L69 3BX

London University

Charing Cross and Westminster Medical School, St Dunstan's Road, London W6 8RP.

King's College Hospital Medical School, Denmark Hill, London SE5 8RX.

The London Hospital Medical College, Turner Street, London E1 2AD.

Royal Free Hospital School of Medicine, Rowland Hill Street, London NW3 2PF.

St Bartholomew's Hospital Medical College, West Smithfield, London EC1A 7BE.

St George's Hospital Medical School, Cranmer Terrace, London SW17 0RE.

St Mary's Hospital Medical School (a constituent College of Imperial College of Science, Technology and Medicine), Norfolk Place, London W2 1PG.

United Schools of Guy's and St Thomas's Hospitals, London Bridge, London SE1 9RT.

University College School of Medicine, Gower Street, London WC1E 5BT.

Medical School, University of Manchester, Oxford Road, Manchester M13 9PT.

Medical School, University of Newcastle, Newcastle upon Tyne NE1 7RU.

Medical School, University of Nottingham, Queen's Medical Centre, Nottingham NG7 2UH.

Medical School, Oxford University, Oxford OX2 6HG.

Medical School, University of Sheffield, Sheffield S10 2TN.

Faculty of Medicine, The University, Southampton SO9 5NH.

Faculty of Medicine, Queen's University, Belfast BT7 1NN.

Faculty of Medicine, University of Aberdeen, Marischal College, Aberdeen AB9 1AS.

Medical School, University of Dundee, Dundee DD1 4HN.

Medical School, University of Edinburgh, Edinburgh EH8 9YL.

Faculty of Medicine, University of Glasgow, Glasgow G12 8QQ.

Faculty of Science, University of St Andrews, St Andrews, Fife.

University of Wales College of Medicine, Heath Park, Cardiff CF4 4XN.

Appendices

Addresses of professional and specialty organisations

College of Anaesthetists, 35–43 Lincoln's Inn Fields, London WC2A 3PN.

Faculty of Public Health Medicine of the Royal Colleges of Physicians of the United Kingdom, 28 Portland Place, London W1N 4DE.

Faculty of Occupational Medicine (see Physicians)

Medical Research Council, 20 Park Crescent, London W1N 4AL.

Royal College of General Practitioners, 14 Prince's Gate, London SW7 1PU.

Royal College of Obstetricians and Gynaecologists, 27 Sussex Place, London NW1 4RG.

Royal College of Pathologists, 2 Carlton House Terrace, London SW1Y 5AF.

Royal College of Physicians, 11 St Andrew's Place, London NW1 4LE.

Royal College of Physicians of Edinburgh, 9 Queen Street, Edinburgh EH2 1JQ.

Royal College of Physicians and Surgeons of Glasgow, 234–42 St Vincent Street, Glasgow G2 5RJ.

Royal College of Psychiatrists, 17 Belgrave Square, London SW1X 8PG.

Royal College of Radiologists, 38 Portland Place, London W1N 3DG.

Royal College of Surgeons of Edinburgh, 18 Nicholson Street, Edinburgh EH8 9DW.

Royal College of Surgeons of England, 35–43 Lincoln's Inn Fields, London WC2A 3PN.

Armed forces medical services:

RAMC Officer Recruiting Team, Regimental Headquarters RAMC, Royal Army Medical College, Millbank, London SW1P 4RJ.

The Medical Director General (Naval), (Attention Med P1(N)), Ministry of Defence, First Avenue House, 40–48 High Holborn, London WC1V 6HE.

Ministry of Defence MA1 (RAF), First Avenue House, 40–48 High Holborn, London WC1V 6HE.

Index

Index

Index